CAUSE

CURE

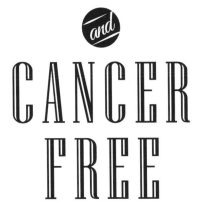

and

CANCER FREE

HOW I BECAME A CANCER ESCAPEE

JOHN MARRA

SAKURA PUBLISHING
Hermitage, Pennsylvania
USA

CAUSE, CURE

AND

CANCER FREE

HOW I BECAME A CANCER ESCAPEE

JOHN MARRA

Sakura Publishing
PO BOX 1681
Hermitage, PA 16148
www.sakura -publishing.com

ORDERING INFORMATION:
Quantity sales: Special discounts are available on quantity purchases by corporations,
associations, and others. For details, contact the publisher at the address above. Orders by
U.S. trade bookstores and wholesalers. Please contact Sakura Publishing:
Tel: (330) 360-5131; or visit
www.sakura-publishing.com.
Book Cover and Interior Design by Rania Meng
Edited by Derek Vasconi

First Edition
Printed in the United States of America
ISBN-13: 978-0-9911807-5-2
ISBN-10: 0991180755

TABLE OF CONTENTS

DISCLAIMER

This publication is intended to provide helpful and informative material. It is not intended to diagnose, treat, cure, or prevent any health problem or condition, nor is it intended to replace the advice of a physician. No action should be taken solely on the contents of this book. Always consult your physician or qualified healthcare professional on any matters regarding your health and before using any suggestions in this book or drawing inferences from it.

The author and publisher specifically disclaim all responsibility for any liability, loss or risk, personal or otherwise, which is incurred as a consequence, directly or indirectly, from the use of applications of any contents of this book.

Any and all product names referenced within this book are the trademarks of their respective owners. None of these owners have sponsored, authorized, endorsed, or approved this book. Always read all information provided by the manufacturers' product labels before using their products. The author and publisher are not responsible for claims made by manufacturers. The statements made in this book have not been evaluated by the Food and Drug Administration.

Some names have been changed to protect the privacy of the individuals discussed within this book.

DEDICATION

FOR NANCY CALAFATO MARRA, MY AMAZING WIFE.

YOU ARE MY RIB.

"The only thing not possible is that which is not imaginable"

JOHN MARRA

Chapter One

For those rusty on their Bible studies, I would like to remind you that the literal meaning of "Gospel" is "good news;" it was the mission of the Apostles to spread the good news of the Lord.

THE FIRST BIG, UNNERVING BLOW hit me while I was standing over the toilet.

It seemed, as I reflected on the past handful of years, that the stress had been accumulating like a snowball down a hill. I'd dealt with the untimely loss of my brother in a motorcycle accident. I'd sold my very lucrative construction business, glad to be rid of the strain it placed on my shoulders, only to find myself the owner of a small, failing radio station that was practically hemorrhaging money. My wife Nancy, a political activist, had just had her email account hacked by an opposition "hacktivist." And to top it all off, the IRS had just decided I was due for an audit.

To think, I had gone out that night to get away from it all.

As devout Catholics, Nancy and I are proud members of Legatus, an organization that helps folks like us spread the message of faith. At the dinner following that night's meeting, I'd sought refuge from my constant tensions with a hearty meal. I helped myself to a generous portion of chicken, chased it with two cocktails—I believe they were vodka cranberries—and didn't say "when" until after I'd finished dessert.

Contented with my king's feast, Nancy and I returned home. In a way, that evening was like every other in recent memory; I'd awaken several times throughout the night with a pressing urge to use the bathroom. But this particular occasion was something else. As I leaned over the toilet to void my bladder, I found myself firing out pure crimson blood. This, as you can imagine, really put the fear of God in me.

Albeit on a much smaller scale, I'd dealt with this sort of thing before. For too long, urination had been an increasingly irritating process, complete with a little pink discoloration here and there. It had even begun to interfere in my relations with my wife. My concern was enough that I'd already scheduled an appointment with my urologist, due in another six days. But as this unadulterated blood incident had left me shaken—terrified, to be quite honest—the doctor agreed to address this emergency the very next day.

That was in the summer of 2011. As I look back at that night, I can't help but think of all I didn't know at the time. I didn't know, for example, that shortly thereafter I would be diagnosed with aggressive Bladder Cancer. I had no idea then that professional medicine's treatment for such a disease promised to rob me of my dignity and my manhood, with no guarantee that any of it would actually cure me.

Of course, it was that very same night that I began piecing the larger picture together. It would not be long before I came to appreciate how my seemingly endless stress was fatiguing my physical body to the point that, in a sense, I'd invited disease upon myself. It would also not be long before I would begin to understand the critical role diet would play in my journey towards healing; I'd quickly learn that in overfeeding myself with all the wrong foods, I was likewise feeding my cancer.

I'd soon come to understand that I had given myself this illness, and that with a better understanding of the problem, a lot of resolve, and endless faith, I could also cure myself more effectively than any traditional medical treatment.

For those rusty on their Bible studies, I would like to remind you that the literal meaning of "Gospel" is "good news;" it was the mission of the Apostles to spread the good news of the Lord. So too am I on a mission to share all I've discovered. While many would consider a cancer diagnosis a death knell, I am grateful for the experience. It has made me wiser, stronger, and as I continue to put into practice the lessons I've learned, a perfectly healthy man to this day. All of this puts me in an ideal position to teach others how to do what I've done—to give them the information they need eat healthfully, conquer tension, and heal themselves.

I know it all seems daunting. What can any person in today's world really do to rid himself of stress? How do we avoid the endless temptations of foods that taste good, but ravage our bodies? We might even suspect that cancer and other chronic ailments are but the unavoidable price we must pay for our toil and our dinners. But the goal of this book is to demonstrate to you, the reader, how to find a place of peace, devoid of the stresses that wear us down. The goal is to tell you of the foods that bring illness upon us—an innumerable amount, believe me—and detail an alternative diet that primes the body for healing and wellness. The goal is to arm you with all the same knowledge that helped me fight and win my battle with cancer.

I don't pretend to be a medical professional. I'm simply a man who stared death in the face, and, unwilling to waver, educated himself, took action, and beat his death sentence. I am very much alive today, and it would be criminal of me to squander that gift of life without teaching others of my path to wellness.

To those who are sick, and for whom traditional medicine holds little hope; to those who long for any solace from the stresses and strains of modern life; to those who wish to eat their way towards health and recovery—I implore you to read on as I share my gift with you.

Chapter Two

"Just don't eat it." He didn't seem at all concerned. I, on the other hand, was certain there was more to it than the doctor was letting on.

I WAS BORN IN CLEVELAND, OHIO into an Italian family with all the traditional values and quirks you'd expect. Our Catholic faith was integral, and our personal exchanges could sometimes get heated. The food I was raised on too should come as no surprise to those familiar with Italian culture; our supply of pasta seemed endless, as did other carbohydrate-rich foods such as cereals and breads.

It was in early adulthood that I began my career in construction. A few short years later, I married my incredible wife Nancy. She was also of Italian heritage, and every evening, as I would come home having worked up a hearty appetite from a long day on the job, she'd have a savory meal at the ready. In addition to the grains I'd grown up with, we dined on all sorts of meat dishes as well—beef, chicken, and meatballs would find their way to our plates just about every night.

I had no idea then the sort of damage these rich foods were doing to my body.

It was in the summer of 2011 that my issues with urination became problematic to the point that I'd scheduled an appointment with my urologist. What began as a simple tingling sensation as I voided—and it seemed that I always had that urge to go—had turned into full-fledged irritation, complete with pink tinges of blood.

As you might recall from the previous chapter, I'd been watching the days tick past, waiting for my visit with the urologist, when I'd indulged at that Legatus dinner only to come home and expel unadulterated blood into the toilet. My appointment was hastened to the following day.

Even early on, I had made some connections between the foods I'd been eating and the resulting irritation. I thought back to one morning in particular when the blood content in my urine had been unusually plentiful—and elimination especially painful. *What did I eat last night?* I asked myself. It had been a few too many bowlfuls of a popular, cocoa-flavored cereal. I grabbed the box and examined its list of ingredients; Red Dye 40 seemed to leap out at me. It began as a simple hunch, but sure enough, every time I ate something containing this red dye, my symptoms would get worse.

Of course I made mention of this to the urologist, who replied simply and tersely: "Just don't eat it." He didn't seem at all concerned. I, on the other hand, was certain there was more to it than the doctor was letting on. *What is this Red Dye 40, anyway? Why might it be causing my inflammation?*

I later did a bit of research, and the answer I found was alarming. FD&C Red 40 is a coloring agent used in all sorts of commercial foods; you'd have to make a real effort to avoid it at the supermarket. Its chemical makeup is 2-naphthalenesulfonic acid, 6-hydroxy-5-((2-methoxy-5-methyl-4-sulfophenyl)azo)-, disodium salt, and disodium 6-hydroxy-5-((2-methoxy-5-methyl-4-sulfophenyl)azo)-2-naphthalenesulfonate. How appetizing does that sound? What's worse, the stuff is made from petroleum, not so different from gasoline. Europe has discouraged children from eating it, while some countries have banned it altogether. Despite protests, Red Dye 40 has been approved by the FDA, and we in the United States are free to eat as much of it as we please.

If the urologist was aware of any of this, he apparently didn't care enough to share it with me. Instead, he adhered to procedure and subjected me to a cystoscopy; this is when a camera on the end of a tube is jammed into the urethra and snaked into the bladder so that the doctor might have a look inside. I'll spare the reader the grisly details—men in particular might find themselves cringing—but suffice it to say, the whole thing hurt like the dickens. It was as if a pipe five inches in diameter had been crammed into a hole half an inch wide.

"Well, I see the polyps," the doctor said nonchalantly. "No big deal," he continued, "we'll zap them out of there, and you're done." The following week after the cystoscopy, he went on to perform a transurethral resection for bladder tumor, or TURBT. With a resectoscope now lodged deep into my bladder, he scraped off the polyps for a biopsy and burned away whatever potentially cancerous tissue that remained.

In a matter of days, the results of the biopsy were ready, and I learned my diagnosis: stage 1 cancer of the bladder. The time had come to see an oncologist.

The doctor I would be visiting at the Cleveland Clinic had a fine reputation, and in regards to Bladder Cancer, the man was supposedly without peer. But as if the urologist's cystoscopy hadn't been a humiliating enough torture, I would quickly discover that the oncologist's treatment of choice—indeed, the method preferred by the entire medical establishment—would be far worse. Their endgame would be a radical cystectomy, or RC. They plotted to remove my bladder, lymph nodes, prostate, and a good four feet of intestines. From this tissue, they would construct a new or "neo" bladder, which would be totally incontinent. The rest of my life would be spent wearing diapers and attending to catheters, with no hope of ever being intimate with my wife again. I'd nevertheless have to go through chemotherapy and radiation, and to top it all off, none of this could guarantee that the cancer wouldn't eventually return.

I wasn't about to accept my diagnosis as a death sentence. But what the doctors had in store for me didn't seem all that much better. There I was, a man in his early fifties, and modern medicine could do no better than to essentially reduce me to an enfeebled 80 year old. I resolved then and there to find another solution.

Much of my time then was spent both in research and in prayer—believe you me, I asked for the Lord to grant me the Wisdom of Solomon so that I might find a way to heal myself. Those prayers, it seemed, did not go unheard, as answers began to trickle forth. Fittingly enough, one of those answers came to me during Mass.

No matter the circumstances of my life, I never failed to attend a church service. On one occasion in particular, I was privy to a reading from the Book of Daniel. Daniel and his men, it seemed, had found themselves in the service of King Nebuchadnezzar of Babylon. So that the men might remain fit to serve, they were instructed to eat from the Kings table; this included all manner of decadent royal meats and wines. But Daniel protested, insisting that for ten days, he and his companions would eat only vegetables and drink only water. After ten days had elapsed, it was clear that Daniel and his group had become perfectly fit physical specimens, with unequalled intellect to boot.

It was hard not to consider it a sign.

I had already made the connection between a food additive like Red Dye 40 and the exacerbation of my symptoms. It made sense that this and similar harmful chemicals could only be avoided through a diet just like Daniel's—water and organic vegetables free from modern pesticides. I had asked my urologist what sort of foods a man with my diagnosis should be eating, to which he replied, "Whatever you want." But as if the Scripture hadn't made it obvious enough that the doctor was dead wrong, I would quickly find enthusiastic affirmation of the power of the "Daniel diet" in two highly esteemed authors and a holistic healer. With their help, I would soon discover that the root of my problem was a condition known as acidosis—and that clean, organic vegetables would be crucial to my recovery.

Chapter Three

"Please test your servants for ten days. Let us be given vegetables to eat and water to drink.

Then see how we look in comparison with the other young men who eat from the royal table, and treat your servants according to what you see."

He agreed to this request, and tested them for ten days;

after ten days they looked healthier and better fed than any of the young men who ate from the royal table.

So the steward continued to take away the food and wine they were to receive, and gave them vegetables.

To these four young men God gave knowledge and proficiency in all literature and wisdom, and to Daniel the understanding of all visions and dreams.

DANIEL 1:12-17   NEW AMERICAN BIBLE (USCCB)

NANCY AND I would often enjoy thick, savory cuts of beef, ground chuck wadded up into meatballs, and, on our occasional efforts to be more "health-conscious," lighter meats such as chicken. We'd take our turns sampling every manner of pasta you could imagine—spaghetti, of course, rigatoni, ravioli, and so many more—all of it packed with starches and made from bleached, enriched grains. And then there were the cheeses, rich dairy delights like Parmesan and Romano. With indulgences such as these weighing down our dinner plates, why wouldn't a glass or two of red wine be in order?

But all of that was before my cancer diagnosis, and well before I'd made the connection between processed foods and the irritation I'd been suffering. And, in light of my revelation at Mass, it was just the sort of sinful fare that the pagan King Nebuchadnezzar would help himself to heartily—but on which wise Daniel would pass. Some might chalk it up to coincidence, but I felt as if I'd been witness to signs, pointing the way to a possible recovery.

I thought of my cancer, and the solutions proposed by every doctor I'd consulted. They'd want to rip me open, leave me wearing diapers, and subject me to the twin traumas of chemotherapy and radiation. All of this would only guarantee that I would be living like an invalid—should I wind up living very long at all. Indeed, according to the pamphlets the oncologist had been kind enough to hand me, the success rates for the radical cystectomy he'd proposed were hardly impressive—after five years, just slightly over a third survive. If the cancer has spread, that number gets even slimmer. In fact, even for those who have undergone such "gold glove" treatments as radiation and chemo, various forms of cancer still claim some 1,600 lives in the United States every day. None of this information left me feeling encouraged.

I found myself going through a kind of long, dark night of the soul. My Bladder Cancer was not likely to just disappear on its own—some kind of treatment was in order, or I'd be staring down certain death. At the same time, the treatments my doctors had devised seemed just as hopeless. Was I willing to take the gamble and live as a kind of half-man, robbed of all vigor and zest for life? What if, as the statistics seemed to indicate, the cystectomy, chemotherapy, and radiation would prove ineffective? Would I wind up spending my last living days in misery for nothing?

My diagnosis was like a gun to the head that had me frantically scrambling for answers. I began to search the cancer support forums online. There I found confirmation that I'd been right to do away with chemical additives like Red Dye No. 40. But as I soon learned, conscientious and informed eaters have far more than just that to avoid at the grocery store. It wasn't long before I became familiar with a condition known as *acidosis*.

On a scale from 0 to 14, every healthy mammal (everything from human beings to rats) should have a pH of around 7; that would be the point of equilibrium between bodily acids and bases. Acidosis refers to the state of having too much acidic content in the blood and tissue, and this condition can set the stage for even further health issues. As my pH testing confirmed, all of those meats, starches, dairy foods, and alcoholic beverages had been throwing off my alkaline-to-acid balance, leaving me vulnerable to all sorts of illnesses. Severe metabolic acidosis, for example, can produce the same effects as ethylene glycol poisoning. In other words, for all the damage those rich Italian foods had done to me, I might as well have been drinking antifreeze.

Again I saw that nightmarish vision of me standing over the toilet the night of that Legatus dinner, and found myself dwelling on just what that incident implied about the connection between wellness and diet. I was hesitant to let myself so much as complete the thought—who was I to question my doctors?—but, desperate for a third alternative, it came to me: *if eating the*

wrong foods has left me in this sickly state, shouldn't eating the right
foods reverse the course of my illness and steer me back to health? If
acidosis is the underlying cause and the cancer just a symptom, shouldn't
I just eat my way to an alkalized state?

I was already fairly well-versed in what all the wrong foods
were; indeed, darned near everything we find ourselves eating in
present-day America contributes to acidosis, leaving us ordinary
folks prone to diabetes, arthritis, and yes, cancer. If my trouble
was having too much acid in my system, it made sense that I had
to increase my alkaline to attain balance. Had anyone else tried
this sort of nutrition-based approach to correcting pH? Could
such a thing reverse the progression of disease?

Sadly, this is not the sort of thing you're likely to hear from
an oncologist, but there are indeed two contemporary practi-
tioners of medicine who have successfully treated people like
me using diets meant to alkalize the system, making their bodies inhospitable to cancer. Just as I've got to credit the Word of
the Lord for my initial inspiration, I must recognize Dr. Leonard
Coldwell and Dr. Robert O. Young for not only confirming my
hunch, but for spelling out some of the details. Coldwell's *The
Only Answer to Cancer* and Young's *The pH Miracle* series proved to
be invaluable guideposts on my journey. Dr. Coldwell's stance
is that Western medicine typically addresses the symptoms of
various illnesses; so long as the root causes of our ailments are
not corrected, we can only expect disease to return. His treatment strategy involves a radical overhaul of the diet, and he
credits this approach for having saved the lives of over 35,000
patients, many with prognoses worse than mine. Dr. Young, too,
is primarily concerned with eating carefully in order to create
a healthy, alkaline environment in the body. A finer pH balance,
Young claims, better steels a person against all manner of maladies, paving the way toward weight loss, higher energy levels, and
optimum blood sugar. In short, his is a diet meant to foster ideal

health. Contrast that with the predicament I found myself in after a lifetime's worth or red meats, pastas, and cheeses.

It's not as if these two doctors don't have their share of critics; indeed they do, and some can get vitriolic. While both have scores of devout followers who'll attest endlessly to the therapeutic value of their teachings, neither enjoys any endorsements from more "reputable" bastions of medicine such as the American Medical Association or the American Cancer Society. I don't believe that the medical professionals who helm these organizations would dismiss Young's and Coldwell's successes due to some heartless attempt to monopolize health care, favoring dollars over human lives. Rather, the medical establishment is comprised of individuals who've spent years upon years in schooling—a kind of brainwashing, perhaps, that has left them unable to consider any sort of evidence that hasn't been handed to them by their professors. In their quest for education, they may have in fact become a bit narrow-minded.

I don't know what I might have been led to believe had I endured countless years in medical school. The fact is that I was an ordinary man with a grim prognosis, hungry for a solution that would let me live both long and fully. And it was the inspiration I found in the words of Coldwell and Young that led me to conceive of my cancer in an entirely different context. Modern medicine seems to contend that disease is a thing to attack, and their tactics are a bit like those of an army on the defensive. I thought instead of health as a thing to be won. Taking care of myself through smart choices in diet struck me as a bit like building an impenetrable fortress, hardy enough to keep illness from so much as rearing its head.

As I considered all of this, an analogy came to mind. Growing up in an Italian household, I would often help myself to salted tomato slices. Now and again, I would wind up with a canker sore or two on the inside of my mouth. Even as a young man, I knew that there'd be no hope of those sores healing if I kept it up with those irritatingly acidic tomatoes. But if I just abstained for a while, eating things less likely to aggravate those tender little sores, I would be creating an environment in which healing was free to take its course. Cancer is hardly the same as a canker sore, and I don't pretend to have invented a cure for anything. But based on all I'd been through and all I'd read, I decided to take that leap of faith—and yes, veering away from the course outlined by one's oncologist requires a heaping dose of faith—to see if I could heal myself by fostering good health through diet, rather than simply destroying the manifestations of illness.

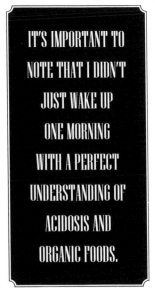

IT'S IMPORTANT TO NOTE THAT I DIDN'T JUST WAKE UP ONE MORNING WITH A PERFECT UNDERSTANDING OF ACIDOSIS AND ORGANIC FOODS.

I'd guessed at the sort of foods I would have to do away with; you don't often hear of anyone extolling the health benefits of red meat. But I was a bit surprised to learn that, given my weakened state, I would have to take supposedly healthier meats like fish and poultry off the menu as well— any animal protein whatsoever could only exacerbate my acidosis. The same is true of animal by-products such as eggs and dairy. Enriched or processed foods of any stripe must similarly be eliminated; I said goodbye to white flour and sugar, as well as anything with any ingredients I would need a degree in chemistry just to pronounce.

As far as beverages go, caffeinated drinks like coffee, tea, and soda were off the table, as were all things alcoholic. And just when it seemed that things couldn't get more restrictive, I learned that fruits contribute to acidosis by virtue of their natural sugars. Even some acidic veggies like corn would be too much for a man with my condition.

It's important to note that I didn't just wake up one morning with a perfect understanding of acidosis and organic foods. Like all things worth having in life, winning this knowledge involved some struggle, or at least trial and error. My search began with an online Bladder Cancer advocacy group. At this point, I'd only begun to get my feet wet in terms of diet—still eating meats like chicken and beef, but this time, only of the certified organic variety. As my exploration of the subject deepened, I consulted holistic healer Dr. Todd Pesek. I learned to do away with the meat, and instead began eating from Pesek's palette of good stuff like flax seed oil—and not so good stuff like cottage cheese and other dairy. And again, it was thanks to the work of Drs. Coldwell and Young that I was able to whittle my menu down to only those most healing foods, armed with an appreciation of pH imbalance. My journey toward this point might have been haphazard—and indeed, as my prognosis failed to improve, I questioned myself every step of the way—but in the end, it was a reading from the Old Testament that steeled my resolve. I knew then, finally, which course to take. So what sort of diet was I left with to alkalize my body and regain my health?

Leafy green vegetables and water. Just like the Book of Daniel said.

You might have noticed the loving detail with which I described my old diet of red meats and pasta. Believe me, it had to have taken something like the threat of impending death to tear me away from my lasagna. The idea of having nothing but leafy greens on my plate and simple water in my glass struck me as a necessary sacrifice I would just have to endure. But strangely, it didn't take long before I developed quite the taste for the surprisingly rich world of vegan cuisine. Even better, I quickly found myself feeling better than I had in years, with those aches and discomforts we associate with age simply vanishing.

Which delectable vegetable dishes taught me to not merely

suffer through, but actually embrace the all green approach? And, perhaps most crucial, what became of the tumors in my bladder?

If you'd rather sit down to eat a salad than be fed cytotoxic antineoplastic drugs, read on.

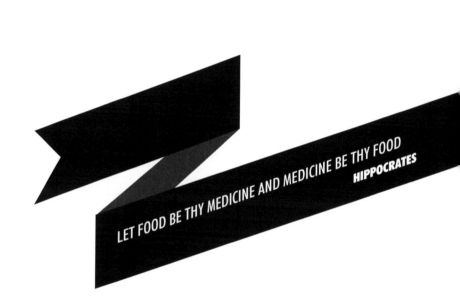

LET FOOD BE THY MEDICINE AND MEDICINE BE THY FOOD

HIPPOCRATES

Chapter Four

THOUGH HONING MY MENU took time to straighten out, I finally undertook the so-called Daniel diet in order to alkalize my body and let healing begin. It seemed simple enough—just stick to green, leafy vegetables. And while such a description would not have steered you wrong in Daniel's day, way back in ancient Babylon, modern man has since made food production a lot more complicated—and a lot less healthy—than things used to be.

Let's take spinach, for example. It's unquestionably a leafy green, and you should have no trouble finding it at just about any supermarket, any time of year. The problem is that most of what's on the shelves is the product of modern industrial farming. As such, we can expect that healthy-looking spinach, and all manner of other produce, to have been treated with chemical pesticides. It's no secret that a bevy of bugs can destroy a farmer's yield. Pesticides aren't by nature a bad thing; for millennia, farmers used a number of natural means to keep insects from ravaging their crops. But around the 20th century, agriculture saw the mass implementation of synthetic pesticides. They can knock swarms of pests dead, and even if we're careful to wash our produce before eating it, it can still find its way into our systems.

When we eat industrial farmed foods, we might find ourselves ingesting roughly thirty different kinds of chemical pesticides—and washing our vegetables first does nothing to get rid of the synthetic toxins that have seeped inside. A great number of studies have confirmed the link between the con-sumption of these pesticides and the development of ailments such as ADHD, Alzheimer's disease, and yes, cancer. Eating these things might not kill us immediately, but as we continue to consume them, they accumulate in our bodies and make us that much more vulnerable to illness. This is especially true in regards to bodily networks such as the endocrine, reproductive, and nervous systems.

Another key drawback about commercially farmed foods is that they are often times subject to irradiation. This is the process by which bacteria is destroyed with blasts of radiation, roughly analogous to the output from millions of X-rays. Not only does this procedure sap foods of their vitamins and nutrients, it also alters their molecular structures. The ionization process gives rise to free radicals, which can bind to the organic materials in food to form formaldehyde, benzene, and other powerful toxins.

But the most dangerous assault yet on otherwise nutritious, healthy produce was introduced in the United States late last century, when genetically modified organisms, or GMOs, became commercially available. In an effort to engineer crops better able to thrive when dosed with pesticides, little strands of DNA, typically from bacteria and viruses, were inserted into the genes of many common vegetables and fruits. As a result, when you sit down to eat something as seemingly innocuous as an apple, you might actually be consuming the genetic information of some microscopic organism that no human in history has ever ingested until recently. Another kind of GMO involves the insertion of genetic code from the bacteria Bacillus Thuringiensis into foods like corn in order to elicit the secretion of biological insecticides. The pests that consume these Frankenstein foods wind up with their stomachs exploding. Their effects on other living things aren't markedly better; since their introduction, allergies to corn and soy (of the genetically modified, or better known as GMO, variety) have increased considerably. Genetically modified foods have been linked to liver malfunction, sterility, and infant mortality in laboratory animals. Livestock the world over have suffered damaged organs and immune systems after eating GMO feed, with vast swaths of animals simply having up and died. None of this would seem to indicate that GMOs are at all safe for human consumption. While such things have been banned outright in nearly every industrialized nation in the world, we in the US have had to wage legal battles just to ensure that genetically modified crops are labeled as such.

It should be obvious at this point why I arrived at a diet of certified organic produce. Organic fare is grown without the use of synthetic fertilizers and chemical pesticides, never subject to irradiation, and untainted by the meddling of genetic scientists. They leave us free to eat as naturally as God intended. But they don't merely spare us from ingesting chemical toxins and spliced bacterial DNA. Organic produce has been shown to contain roughly 50% more antioxidants than foods grown under industrial conditions, and are far richer in vitamins and minerals. Eating them primes the body to fight off cancer and heart disease and strengthens immune function. And if you're the sort, like me, who never used to care much for the taste of vegetables, wait until you savor the rich flavors of organics.

Perhaps if I began adhering to a vegetarian, all-organic diet years ago, I'd have never developed cancer in the first place. I don't doubt that this would have been the case. But the fact of the matter is that I had been eating unhealthily, and I had to meet my cancer diagnosis eye-to-eye. I had to take every precaution, and as I'd soon learn, that would mean paring down my organic diet to something a bit more restrictive. I would absolutely have to eliminate the underlying acidosis that had caused my health issues, and in order to make that happen, I would have to eat only those foods that would return my body to an alkalized state.

If a perfectly healthy person had to choose between eating an apple and eating a cheeseburger, I would of course implore him to opt for the apple—that fruit is the healthier alternative is just common sense. But I was by no means a perfectly healthy person. The hypothesis that the root cause of my problem was acidosis quite obviously implied that acidic foods were off the table; this meant I had to avoid apparently healthy organics like oranges and lemons just as surely as I avoided coffee and vinegar dressings. And though I knew I was in dire straits, I was still a bit surprised to learn that given my weakened state, it wasn't just the citrus I would have to do away with—every fruit imaginable would be off limits. This is because fruits contain a kind of sugar known as fructose. While far healthier for a person than ordinary white sugar, trying to digest any kind of sugar at all can place undue strain on one's system, and a man in my position did not have the luxury of taking any chances. I had to say goodbye to not just the ice-cream and chocolate syrup, but the seemingly healthy fruity toppings as well. The same was true for certain vegetables such as carrots and beets, as those too contained more sugar than my system could handle at the time.

Sugar, as we know, is a simple carbohydrate. But what of the complex carbohydrates such as foods high in fiber? Here was another instance where what might have been permissible for a fellow in good health would have been too much for me. We're all likely familiar with the marathon runner's habit of "carbo-loading" the night before a run. The idea here is that these densely-packed carbohydrates make for a slow digestive burn, providing a steady release of energy for the runner throughout the following day. This, as it turns out, was exactly the sort of thing I had to avoid. Complex carbohydrates—including the fibrous plant and grain material we're advised to eat for digestive health—would have been a real chore to digest, placing even more stress on my vulnerable system. Remember that the point of this exercise was to promote healing; a body taxed by strenuous efforts to process fiber cannot recuperate effectively.

It might seem as if I'd taken essentially everything worth eating off the menu. But I was hardly left staring at an empty plate. Far from it; this endeavor introduced me to a new world of culinary creations that I might never have explored otherwise. Leafy greens include everything from alfalfa to wheatgrass, with stops along the way for cucumbers, kale, broccoli, asparagus, and so much more. Roasting such veggies, or frying them up in a bit of extra virgin olive oil, is a real treat I have come to look forward to. But to unlock the benefits of these organic goods to maximum effect, I took to juicing.

Juicers range from the relatively inexpensive to the higher-end luxury models. Regardless of the price, it's important that your juicer has both fines blades to mince your vegetable material, as well as a system for funneling the fibrous cell exteriors away from the nutrition locked away inside those cells. Vitamins, minerals, and essential phytonutrients make their way into the juice, while the pulpy fiber—the sort of thing that makes our digestive systems work overtime—is discarded. In this way, juicing delivers the most nutritive, nourishing parts of the plant in a way that the body can handle effortlessly. And yes, a nice wheatgrass smoothie is yet another of the many veggie delights I've developed quite a taste for.

As I proceeded with my diet—still working out the kinks at this point, but learning more every day—I'd noticed that I no longer had to urinate as frequently or as urgently as I once did, and the irritation had all but vanished. The true test would come when I steeled my resolve, did my best to banish any lingering fears, and set off for the Cleveland Clinic for another cystoscopy.

The oncologist explained to me that this procedure would again involve the insertion of a tiny camera into my bladder. While observational in nature, the doctor remarked that, should any new cancerous material be discovered, it would be removed and sent to the pathology department. I was confident, however, that my diet could have only improved the situation.

I should not have to remind the reader—men in particular—of what a painful ordeal my first cystoscopy had been. This time, I insisted on being anaesthetized. To put it bluntly, they knocked me out. I awoke some time later to find Nancy sobbing by my bedside.

"They found four new tumors," she tearfully told me, "even bigger than the first ones."

CHAPTER FOUR

Quite frankly, I was floored. I'd followed my diet to the best of my understanding. Had I been barking up the wrong tree? Was it time to give up and subject myself to a radical cystectomy? Would I have to resign myself to a life of incontinence—very likely a brief life at that?

The doctor was adamant that this was indeed my only option. In the time I was out, he'd implored my wife to convince me to undergo his treatments. Nancy, however, knew my fighting spirit full well. Looking out the window on a clear day, she gestured to the man-made marvels surrounding the clinic.

"Look at these buildings," she'd said to him. "Do you think they were built by calm followers, or anxious leaders? My husband is an anxious leader."

Nancy was right in her assessment. Following the doctors down their unsteady path was not something I was willing to do—I'd sooner forge my own way. I remained certain that healing via organic foods was my only acceptable option. There just had to be some crucial element I was missing, a methodology meant to work in tandem with the organic approach, not in opposition to it. What steps hadn't I taken? How could I bolster the healing effects of a decent diet to the point of full recovery?

As if I hadn't already been through enough, the weight of my latest prognosis placed a huge emotional strain on me. When Nancy described me as an "anxious leader," *anxious* might have been the key word. And then it came to me. If trying to digest the simple fructose in carrots and beets would place undue stress on my system, inhibiting recovery, then what of the profound psychological stresses I'd been enduring?

I would not waver from my dietary approach to healing; instead, I would accentuate it. Just as I'd eliminated foods that were not conducive to recovery, I would have to do some belt-tightening of a different sort. Daunting as it seemed, I soon set out to eliminate every imaginable stress from my life.

"I'm angry at God," I confessed to the priest.

"It's okay," he replied, "He's got big shoulders.
He can take it."

Chapter Five

AS I MIGHT HAVE MADE CLEAR in Chapter One, I'd never been a stranger to stress. Before I was lucky enough to meet Nancy, I'd been through a divorce. I'd endured the untimely passing of my brother, Jimmy. And operating a construction business left me vulnerable to a lawsuit that might have cost me millions. These were but the worst of times; a comprehensive list of all my stresses, like anyone else's, could fill its own book.

I hadn't quite made the connection at the time, but as I look back, it seems that the initial symptoms that brought me to the doctor—namely, frequent, urgent urination marked with irritation and tinges of blood—would intensify during these peak periods of stress. As anyone who's been through a similar ordeal might tell you, a cancer diagnosis can make a person reevaluate just about everything in life. Just as I became newly aware of the mistakes I'd been making with unhealthy foods, my diagnosis put me in a position to think critically about the ways I'd been handling tension and anxiety—no small feat for a hot-blooded Italian like me.

As I began to educate myself, I discovered that there are actually two types of stress, *eustress* and *distress*. Eustress is a good kind of stress, if you can imagine such a thing. It's that pressure that keeps us on our toes and coaxes the best out of us. Think of a star athlete on the spot, with a stadium full of fans egging him on to perform; it's this kind of eustress that compels him to excel. Distress—a term that surely we're all more familiar with—is another matter entirely. It's the sensation we feel when we're faced with trial after trial with no time to regroup or recuperate. We've all had those times when a bit of distress has kept us awake long nights, or interfered with our digestion. But for people like me, who've had no chance to come up for air, leaving these stresses unchecked can do far greater harm to our bodies than we might suspect. In fact, as many as 90% of all calls to the doctor involve ailments that are caused by excess tension. The most common of these are headaches, pain in the chest, and high blood pressure. In my case, all the pressure I'd experienced day in and day out did just as much to feed my cancer as did my inadequate diet.

There is, I learned, an established link between stress and acidosis—and if you'll recall, acidosis was exactly the culprit Robert O. Young held responsible for diseases like my Bladder Cancer. To reiterate from chapters prior, acidosis occurs when the body creates more acid than it has the capacity to eliminate. Highly acidic foods, like simple and complex carbohydrates, are just part of the situation. My tension had been so profound that it actually compromised my immune system and impaired the function of my organs. All of this made me far less capable of ridding my body of those acids that turned my bladder into fertile ground for tumors.

Stress to a degree like mine, or worse, is enough to kill a person in and of itself; the stereotypical overworked character who reacts to bad news with a coronary heart attack is really no joke. And it should be abundantly clear that our supermarkets offer us a million ways or more to eat ourselves into the grave. But overwhelming stress coupled with a poor diet can work like the twin barrels of a shotgun. Each on its own can release a crippling blast, but together, the damage inflicted is doubly extreme.

There is, in the medical literature, a story of a boy whose malnutrition alone would have caused him to develop mild metabolic acidosis; while hardly an enviable condition, taking corrective measures would have been no Herculean task. But quite unfortunately for this poor little boy, he'd also been through some psychological traumas that further inhibited his body's ability to process and eliminate acids. As a result, he developed not just mild but severe metabolic acidosis, landing him in the intensive care unit for days. My heart goes out, of course, to that little soldier.

It's important to note that in this child's case, his malnutrition was due to outright starvation. Now, no one might have guessed that I myself was starving in any way, shape, or form. I certainly wouldn't have. But as I learned, we in the United States have developed a curious new way to put on the pounds and still be undernourished. Take a look at the snack aisle at your local grocer and you'll see what I mean: we have at our disposal an endless supply of processed foods that offer too much in the way of calories, and virtually nothing in the way of actual nutrition. We might not consider ourselves a nation of starving people, but just like that dear little child, too many of us are getting next to nothing of substance from our diets. I certainly hadn't been. And just like him, the unending stress I'd undergone, combined with my lack of genuine nourishment, had resulted in toxic levels of acid in my blood and tissue.

The notion of launching dual assaults on poor diet and tension to correct my acidosis eventually became clear, thanks in large part to my explorations in alternative medicine. But things weren't always so cut and dry. I'd pressed ahead with an increasingly restrictive diet in hopes of avoiding that radical cystectomy. And on that day when the oncologist reported finding four new, aggressive tumors in my bladder, I had to ask myself quite honestly whether my whole dietary effort had been a failure. Perhaps the alternatives—incontinence at best, an early grave at worst—were still too much to even consider. But for whatever reason, I decided that, far from giving up, I had to press ahead *even further*. The acidosis that had rendered me ill had two great underlying causes: poor dietary choices and stress. There could be no resolving one without addressing the other. A half-hearted approach would not be enough; I would have to eat healthily and eliminate stress, and do so 100%.

Previous chapters describe the foods on which I'd come to thrive in some detail; my footing was not always steady, and it took some time to perfect this diet. Learning to do away with all the tension I could would be a similarly haphazard journey. I began by avoiding those little annoyances that can sour a person's day. As so many of us know, driving a car can invite all manner of frustrations—accidents, road rage, blown tires, or even just the simple but infuriating experience of getting cut off in traffic. I was very fortunate in that Nancy, my wife and my rock, was able to assume command of the wheel. She may have babied me a bit here, but my dire situation called for such measures. The sheer act of riding in the passenger seat, relatively unconcerned with the road, went a long way towards restoring my peace.

Like so many others today, I'd also been a bit of a news junky. It seemed the television was always tuned to the cable news channel, where at any given moment, day or night, I could watch the latest catastrophe unfold at home or abroad. It seems we're all compelled to stay informed of current events, but gone are the days of Walter Cronkite spending just one hour an evening filling us in on the essentials; the 24 hour news cycle can seem like an unending litany of horrors. A story about the nitwits in Washington might leave me fuming, or a piece about the latest terrorist threat might leave me petrified. Whatever the headlines, it seemed they could only put me on edge. It was then that I summoned a power we've all got within, but for too many of us, the thought never crosses our minds—I simply grabbed the remote, hit the "off" button, and learned to appreciate the silence.

I don't know a working person alive who hasn't come home after a long day only to indignantly declare, "I need a vacation!" But the chances for such things, and the means to make them happen, seem to come along too rarely; often the closest we get is when we fix ourselves a stiff drink before bed. Just as I've been lucky to have a wife like Nancy there to chauffeur me around, I was similarly blessed to have the time and resources to vacation in idyllic Florida. On my own, unconcerned with hassles like taking the kids to Disneyworld, I was free to relax and watch the stress just drain away. But I'm fully aware that for the majority of people, rides and vacations can be unimaginable luxuries. Even though I wasn't free to spend every possible minute living carefree on the beach, I'd discovered a path toward peace readily available to everyone, wealthy, struggling, or even destitute. And for me, this did more to eradicate tension than any holiday retreat ever could.

Salvation is a thing for which no person should have to hand over a dollar. I'd been raised Catholic, and have cherished my faith throughout my life. I have to admit that, upon my diagnosis, I was shaken to the point that I questioned just about everything. In other words, I was no longer in a healthy relationship with God. I felt betrayed. *Why me?* I asked. *Haven't I always been your humble servant?* Despite my misgivings, I never wavered from my regular attendance at Mass. It was during confession one day that I mustered the courage to reveal what seemed to me like a Cardinal Sin.

"I'm angry at God," I confessed to the priest.

"It's okay," he replied, "He's got big shoulders. He can take it."

With that, I realized that the powerful shoulders of the Lord would always make for steady ground to stand on—and suddenly, I found that my own shoulders were a bit less tense. The act of confession was not simply a chore in which I prattled off my transgressions; rather, it was a great unburdening. Whatever issues had been eating me up inside had been externalized, and I was free to move on with a lighter heart.

For those whose faiths do not entail the tradition of confession, I imagine that visiting a therapist provides a similar avenue by which to get things off one's chest. And for some, this might be all a person needs. But I don't know of any licensed counselor who can honestly offer what the Lord has given me—sanctifying grace. That is, confession isn't just a matter of verbalizing our woes. It's the process of inviting God's forgiveness, and with that comes the resolve to abstain from such offenses again. This grace fashions the soul into a more perfect thing, less concerned about feelings of guilt and unworthiness. Ask any Catholic—we seem to feel guilt to an almost crippling degree. The notion that God has forgiven me, and I'd in turn become a better person, was like having a yoke lifted off of my back. This, as you might imagine, eliminated more stress than a lifetime's worth of Florida vacations.

I would never dare suggest that Catholicism is about sinning, confessing, and calling it a day. We strive for righteousness, but with this must come a healthy dose of humility. We are asked to walk humbly with our Lord, and Jesus, as we know, was no draconian dictator. He dined with prostitutes and healed lepers—those folks that the Pharisees considered "untouchable." He did this in part to demonstrate that each and every one of us, no matter our mistakes, can still be redeemed. As we walk in the footsteps of Christ, we are urged to forgive others, no matter the degree to which they've hurt or betrayed us. Like confession, practicing forgiveness can lighten the soul in wondrous ways. To cling to resentment is to be stuck in a stasis, with no avenue by which we can grow personally or spiritually. But as we forgive others, we'll find ourselves unshackled, free to move on. There aren't words enough for me to describe just how liberating it has been for me to release all bitterness and let the past be the past. If confession let me loose from my yoke, forgiving others allowed me to walk on air, as the stresses that festered inside of me simply dried up.

So I'd learned that I could eat nothing but lettuce and still never hope to recover; to address the acidosis that impaired my bodily function and threatened my life, I would have to rid myself of potentially deadly stresses as well. For those who've been blessed as I have, time to oneself on a vacation getaway is ideal for melting away tension. But for those who'd have to squirrel away loose change for years just to afford such a thing, there's another answer, and it might be the most powerful of all. Calming the agitated soul is an integral part of healing. For those less spiritually inclined, it might be a matter of talking to a health care professional, or learning to move past old traumas and resentments. For me, it meant inviting the forgiveness of the Lord, and offering that same sort of forgiveness to all those who'd ever left me slighted. Either way, the end result should be a newfound peace great enough to supplant any feelings of tension.

As I'd sat there groggy on that hospital bed, hearing my condition had only worsened, I was tempted to give up on my diet of all leafy greens. Instead, I made up my mind to buttress my organic menu with an effort to shake the stress that had held me down. I knew I would have to give it my all, or the whole endeavor would amount to nothing. I also knew full well that I was taking a gamble, and the stakes could not have been higher.

It was in April, 2012 that I returned to the oncologist for another cystoscopy. The Daniel diet I eventually arrived at left me feeling better than I had in some time, and there was no question that my faith-based approach to eliminating stress had unburdened my spirit immeasurably. But had it been enough to save my life?

The answer was in the doctor's icy hands.

Chapter Six

IT TOOK A BIT MORE than just trial and error. After all, I hardly
had the luxury of fumbling around, seeing what failed and what
succeeded. I'd been diagnosed with aggressive Bladder Cancer;
I could have very conceivably lost my life, and traditional medicine's proposed alternative didn't seem much more appealing. I
deliberately set out to educate myself as best as I could regarding less conventional therapies—it was Drs. Coldwell, Young,
and Pesek, of course, who provided me with the platform from
which I began my trek toward recovery. It started with a keener
awareness of the sort of foods I would have to avoid, and evolved
into a rigid menu featuring a virtual pharmacopeia of leafy
green vegetables. Along the way, I learned that the elimination
of stress was just as integral as the healthiest of diets, and here,
too, I could not afford to compromise. All of it was an effort to
neutralize the acidosis that fed the tumors within, based on the
pretense that this would steer me back to wellness. Still, this
uncharted ground was like walking a tightrope; I had to summon
the strength to keep moving forward, and the faith that I would
make it to the other side.

After I'd worked out the kinks, I spent a few weeks adhering to the Daniel diet and asking the Lord to bring peace to
my heart. But even though I learned to love my leafy greens, it
wasn't a walk in the park. I began to feel a bit of nausea, and a
few aches and pains here and there. This might have been daunting had I not known enough to brace for it. I was in the process of cleansing my body, and all of the toxins I'd accumulated
throughout the years were working their way out of my system.
Discomfort is to be expected as these poisons have their last hur-
rah before finally burning up. But I would have to describe it all
as a *good* kind of pain, much the same way that the rough hands of
a masseuse can tease a dull ache into a feeling of relaxation. Not
only did these minor but unpleasant sensations subside in time,
but gradually, I began to urinate far less frequently, and with far

less urgency. Gone were the symptoms that brought me to the doctor in the first place.

After three months of this, I had a feeling I had done something right. But there was only one way to be sure. I phoned the doctor, and scheduled another cystoscopy.

My first experience with a scope was traumatic enough that I'd insisted that I be good and knocked out for my second. This time, however, I wanted to be wide awake, my eyes fixed on the screen, waiting anxiously to see if my efforts had paid off. In glaring contrast to that nightmarish initial cystoscopy, this occasion was surprisingly bearable. It made sense that, if my symptoms had diminished or disappeared outright, then my tissue should be far less inflamed and sensitive. I would never call having a camera snaked up the urethra a good time, but this lack of abject pain seemed like an indication that I had healed up to an appreciable degree.

There was the image on the monitor, broadcasted straight from within my bladder. **Not a tumor in sight.** The only remarkable features I saw at all were three faint blotches, which looked to me just like new, pink skin in the process of healing over.

I was elated. My efforts had not been in vain—far from it. Whereas once the contents of my bladder threatened to be the death of me, taking command of my diet and stress levels seemed to have eradicated those tumors better than any radical cystectomy could.

The doctor was not so enthusiastic. While he acknowledged that on the whole, there had been an astounding improvement, he voiced his concern about those little pink marks. He told me they could be carcinoma in situ—cancer in its beginning stages—and offered to perform another biopsy.

With that scope in his hand, I was half tempted to tell him where to stick it. Instead, I politely declined his offer. I'd seen too much in the way of confirmation that my method had worked. I resolved to continue to live stress-free and eat only leafy greens until every last trace of the cancer was certifiably gone.

"When you see me again," I told the doctor, "my bladder will be pristine." In four months' time, I returned, making good on that promise. No tumors, no polyps, no discoloration. My insides were perfectly spotless.

I must stress again that I *do not have* a medical degree hanging on my office wall to glance at smugly should anyone question my authority. I'm one man, as ordinary as the next. But the fact is that the medical establishment found cancerous tissue within me. I explored alternative solutions to the problem, based on the pretense that the underlying cause of my cancer was acidosis. Some of the methodologies I arrived at were told to me explicitly, some I modified to suit my circumstances, and others I happened upon by grace. What matters is that it *worked*—those same doctors who discovered my disease were able to confirm that, after the rigors I'd put myself through, all traces of that disease had vanished. If I was able to heal myself in this fashion, it would make sense that others in similar situations should be able to follow my strategy with similarly successful results. Surgery, chemotherapy, and radiation can take far too much out of a person, and none of these treatments are guaranteed to work. If my approach can spare just one person from both these trials and an early grave, telling my story will have been worth it. With this in mind, we'll explore what worked for me in a bit more detail.

ALKALIZING ORGANIC VEGETABLES INCLUDE:

CHAPTER SIX

{ A }

ALFALFA
ASPARAGUS

{ B }

BARLEY GRASS
BROCCOLI
BRUSSELS SPROUTS

{ C }

CABBAGE
CELERY
COLLARD GREENS
CUCUMBERS

{ G }

GARLIC
GINGER

{ K }

KALE

{ L }

LETTUCE

{ M }

MUSTARD GREENS

{ S }

SPINACH
SPROUTS

{ W }

WHEAT GRASS
WILD GREENS

{ Z }

ZUCCHINI

Remember that the issue at hand, in cases like mine and many others, was always acidosis—again, an imbalance in my body's pH that left me susceptible to the development of cancer. The excess acids in my system had robbed my cells of oxygen and nutrients, and impeded the repair of damaged tissue. Healing could only begin if I returned my body to a more alkaline state. In terms of diet, it was acidic food that got me into this mess. Just as surely, the most head-on means of correcting the issue was to eat only those foods that restored balance between my bodily acids and bases. To say that I ate only organic, leafy greens narrows the field some, but this might still be a little ambiguous. Any truly comprehensive list of alkalizing vegetables would be too ambitious for the scope of this book; vegetation, after all, is abundant in God's Creation. For all we know, there could be an undiscovered flowering vine growing in the Amazon rainforest that can alkalize the body with just one spoonful, but it's not the sort of thing you'll find at the farmer's market. The list that follows is by nature incomplete, but should be enough to get any person going in the right direction.

To make the point perfectly clear, it's imperative that the above veggies be from a certified organic source. Opening up a can of, say, industrial farmed spinach can be convenient and comparatively cheap. But as we've seen, commercial food production, even when it comes to something so seemingly wholesome as produce, often entails the use of chemical pesticides and fertilizers, antibiotics, and at times, even gene splicing. It took thousands of cases of congenital deformities before the FDA figured out that thalidomide had no place on the market. As each day seems to bring yet another report of the carcinogenic effects of artificial tinkering with our food supply, I can only hope that these toxins too will someday be similarly outlawed. Until that day arrives, organic foods are our only safe bet.

Some attest that fruit is to be a part of any alkalizing diet. But remember that acidosis is not purely the result of the foods we eat, but of physical and emotional stress as well. While not strictly acidic, complex carbohydrates are to be avoided, as the body must expend excess energy just to break them down. So too can simple carbohydrates in the form of fruit sugars place undue strain on the digestive system; when a person's situation is as dire as mine had been, even fructose-rich vegetables like carrots and beets are off the table.

In keeping with the notion of making digestion as painless as possible, I should remind readers that juicing is the ideal means by which to consume this green goodness. As stated previously, the juicing process does away with the tough, fibrous exteriors of the plant cells, leaving only the nutrient-rich insides for consumption. This delivers all of the nourishment locked within, but none of the fiber that would make our bodies work overtime.

I'm often asked what sorts of beverages are permissible on my alkalizing diet. The answer could not be simpler: water. True, decaffeinated green tea from an organic source is forgivable now and then, but to play things perfectly safe, purified H2O is really the only game in town. Ordinary water should have a pH of around 7.0—that is, neither acid nor base, but neutral. But there's a "hack" here that can take this natural hydrating substance even further in terms of reducing acidosis. The addition of one or two ingredients found in nearly every household refrigerator can tip the scales toward the alkaline. The first would be com-mon baking soda, so high in alkaline content that a mere half-teaspoon's worth is enough to turn an entire gallon of water into a powerful rejuvenating serum. If you've been keeping up thus far, the second ingredient should come as a real surprise: fresh lemon. Yes, acidic fruits are to be avoided like the plague, and lemons are among the most acidic of all. But note that we're not talking about prepackaged lemon juice, or even a slice that's been exposed to the open air for more than a half hour. Perfectly fresh lemons are described by chemists as being *anionic*; that is, rich in negatively charged ions. The anions of a fresh lemon, when ingested, react with the body's digestive juices to produce a surplus of alkaline that far outweighs the lemon's initial acidity. Even the healthiest of us are advised to stay well hydrated. For those battling acidosis, purified water with a nicely-mixed dash of baking soda and fresh lemon can flush toxins from the cells and bring the body's pH up to optimal levels.

As discussed in chapters prior, I might have supped upon nothing but pure heavenly nectar without any improvement at all to my acidosis; diet is, in its own way, paramount, but still only half of the story. The stress I'd been shouldering for so many years was just as detrimental to my physical well-being as any GMO meats might have been. I've been as specific as I can in regards to which foods go the furthest in terms alkalizing the body and ridding the tissue of the stuff in which cancer grows. A blueprint for eliminating stress cannot, by nature, be so cut and dry. No two people have identical temperaments, so what might be relaxing fare for one might actually be intolerable for another. Listening to music, for example, is often times cited as a means to sooth the soul. But while Dick might find solace in a tender Beethoven sonata, Jane might settle for nothing other than the rousing punk idealism of the Clash. So too might Dick find great comfort in a springtime stroll through the outdoors, while for Jane, the same thing would simply amount to hay fever. No person can honestly prescribe a point-by-point plan of doing away with tension that works for everyone across the board. Here, too, I can only speak of what worked for me, and implore readers to discern for themselves what best serves their own fretful minds.

I'd mentioned some of those irritants I'd encountered in everyday life that had the propensity to drive me batty. Driving,

for one, had always been a chore at best, beyond irksome at
worst. I was extremely fortunate in that my wife was willing to
take the reins and let me unclench my teeth. Cable television
news, too, was the sort of potentially blood-boiling experience I
would have to do away with. I imagine these things are common
enough—and annoying enough—that suggesting we hand over
the keys and click off the TV should
do a great number of stressed out people some good. But
regardless
of the particulars, we must identify those things that dampen our
spirits, whatever they might be, and do whatever is within reason
to eliminate them.

But what of those things over which we have no control?
Too few of us, for example, can honestly brag about how much
we love our jobs; more likely, we trudge off daily to what must
seem like a necessary evil. Who can really afford to walk away
from workplace stresses when there are bills to be paid? Here
is another sort of instance in which, after all else has failed, it
was faith that kept me moving in the right direction. Christian
doctrine has never been short on wisdom; it's been with us two
thousand years and counting for good reason. Anyone faced with
seemingly insurmountable troubles, regardless of their religious
inclinations, would be well advised to revisit the Serenity Prayer.
For those who need reminded, it goes
as such:

*God, grant me the serenity to accept
the things I cannot change;
the courage to change the things I can;
and the wisdom to know the difference.*

Note here the humility with which we must acknowledge that picking off the ills of the world one by one is beyond the scope of any person. Some things will be forever beyond our reach. We can spend our days crying about it to no end, or we can invite *serenity* into our hearts. The world outside might not change appreciably, but within us, there can be a calm that carries us through the worst.

I've written at length about how Catholicism has always been my rock. While darned near anyone would make a welcome addition to my congregation, the point of this book is not to win converts to the fold. That said, the surest path to peace of mind is to nurture the spirit, whatever that might entail for a given individual. For some, gazing in wonder at a sunset can instill in us a sense of the everlasting. Others might prefer a more traditional religious backdrop, and the sense of acceptance and community this can bring. Still others might find that weekly visits to a therapist can do the trick.

For me, it was the practice of forgiveness that lightened my soul. I'd begged the Lord to forgive my trespasses, and found myself feeling again like a *good* person, free from the shackles of guilt, no matter my imperfections. Just as important, it was only in forgiving others that resentments I'd harbored for years were finally cast aside. As we forgive, we release negativity and become more fully our very best selves. This doesn't necessarily have to be a religious process; even those of little or no faith will feel buoyed when they let past issues recede into the past. Stepping out from behind the wheel and silencing the television were but luxuries. It was in tending to my spirit, asking for redemption, and granting the same to all those I'd encountered that all of my stresses were vanquished. I can think of no better advice for those with anxious hearts.

I've noted that the healthiest diet conceivable can yield no fruit if the acid-producing problem of stress is not addressed.

Some might think the latter is the more important issue of
the two, and calm their tensions while still leaving room for
sodas and potato chips. Simply put, it just doesn't work that
way. Neither approach has a leg to stand on without the other.
Furthermore, with both diet and stress reduction, there can be
no firing at anything less than full throttle. Every facet of the
program I've described must be embraced wholeheartedly. To
waver in the slightest is to invite failure. Believe me, I can tell
you from experience that this is no easy feat. We might think
that after all of the asparagus we've been eating, a little slice of
cheesecake can do no real harm. We might not see the necessity
of practicing calm every time that jerk neighbor lets his dog do
its business on the lawn again. But one must summon the resolve
to stay on course. It was, after all, my very life that was on the
line. I can't imagine there's cheesecake good enough to have let
that slip away from me.

It all began with the news that a cluster of errant cells in my
bladder might be the beginning of the end for me. In my refusal
to accept anything less than a life lived fully, I schooled myself
on all things acidosis. This, I believe, was the issue central to my
well-being, and the cancer but a symptom. I kept hearkening
back to that boyhood insight about the canker sore and tomatoes;
when I figured out enough to stop irritating that tender tissue
with the offending fruit, the body was free to heal of its own
accord. My health problems later in life were not fundamentally
different. In feeding my acidosis through an unhealthy diet and
unchecked stress, I was only aggravating my condition. Just as
I'd done with those salted tomato slices, I would have to abstain
from decadent foods and live without tension before my system
could correct itself. Sure enough, as pH test strips confirmed,
the acids in my body ebbed away.

As I'd said, the whole thing had been quite a gamble. I
might not have been so fortunate; folks might have remarked

about what a noble experiment I'd undertaken, genuflected before my casket, and said their last goodbyes. But the darnedest thing is that it *worked*. No surgeon jabbed his scalpel in me, no chemotherapy robbed me of my hair—and still I am alive, perfectly **cancer free**.

This is the story I have lived to tell. It might not have made the evening news, but I would be remiss not to share it with every person who's got an ear to lend. *Here is what I did*, I say, *and it saved me*.

Some, at this point, have listened to my tale. And as you'll see, I'm no longer the only one who's been saved.

Chapter Seven

I HAD BEATEN CANCER.

It's a strange thing to hear oneself say, to look back at a time when the grisly reaper's sickle was just inches away from my neck—but now all of that is behind me. On the pretense that acidosis was the underlying cause of my ills, I'd adopted a totally organic diet and taken every conceivable measure to live without stress, all in an effort to bring my body into a more alkaline state. Some told me it was a fool's errand, that conventional medicine was the greatest and perhaps only hope I had. But I am certifiably alive and cancer-free. How could I be less than totally convinced that my acidosis hypothesis was correct, and that acting on that hypothesis spared me from the grave?

I'd saved myself, and my reward was good health and the gift of life. This is hardly the sort of thing a man ought to squander. I believe wholeheartedly that I have in my hands a blueprint for wellness—one that wouldn't cost an arm and a leg, or require risky surgeries and medications that pose more harm than good—and it would be my mission to share all I'd learned with others. Remember once more that I conceived of my cancer as being merely symptomatic of a greater disorder. With all the acids that had accumulated in my system, illness was bound to rear its head in some form or another. If my approach was enough to vanquish that which causes cancer, king of all maladies, I wondered—*what other ailments can proper diet and stress elimination ward off?*

My quest began on the small scale, within my home. My wife Nancy, who has always been my unwaveringly faithful partner through my trials, had long suffered from rashes on the skin. In the past handful of years, her condition had gotten such that she'd awaken some days with what looked like baseball-sized welts on her face, neck, arms, and back. She also suffered from asthma and even a case of goiters at one point. But, unwilling to let me go on my healing journey unaccompanied, Nancy too transitioned to an organic, vegan diet. She's been free of her asthma, goiters, and rashes since.

A few more words regarding my wife. The old adage that behind every good man is an even better woman is, in my experience, absolutely true. When the stress of simply driving became too much for me, Nancy grabbed the wheel without complaint. But that was no real ordeal for her compared to watching her husband dangle over the brink. She shouldered quite a bit then, immersing herself in just the sort of tensions I'd tried so hard to avoid. It should have come as no surprise then that, in January of 2012, Nancy discovered a lump in her breast. But when I say that she, too, underwent an alkalizing diet, I don't mean that she simply sampled my dishes now and again while still eating meats and cheeses on the sly. Rather, she went to every last extreme I did, forsaking everything but select leafy greens and water. She even followed along in my juicing regimen. Just as I don't believe the disappearance of my tumors was a mystery unrelated to my diet, I also don't believe it was due to sheer coincidence that, after so much time spent eating mindfully, Nancy's lump eventually vanished.

Then there was the matter of my mother-in-law. She's lived eighty-some years at this point, God bless her, but many of those years were spent suffering from arthritis. Like many older folks, chicken was a regular staple of her diet. Though hesitant to let it go, I convinced her to doing away with meat. Her arthritis is no longer an issue. So too was it that, after imploring her to do away with dairy, the allergies that plagued my mother-in-law through-out her life have vanished.

On one occasion, my mother-in-law, perhaps feeling a bit out of sorts, went into a pharmacy and hastily checked her blood pressure. Noting that her systolic was well over 200—off

the charts—the attending clerks saw to it that she made her
way to urgent care. After arriving in the emergency room, she
was admitted to Cleveland's Hillcrest Hospital for over two
days. Doctors there prescribed her medication that reduced her
systolic blood pressure to a comparatively low but still-more-
than-ideal 140. If the legally mandated disclaimers we see in
advertisements for prescription drugs are any indication, the
side effects of such things are often just as troublesome as the
conditions they're meant to address. This was exactly the case
with my wife's mother. In the two weeks following her discharge,
the pills she received left her delirious—hardly her usual self.
Her head seemed to swim, and she took a tumble four different
times. Falling spells, as we all know, can be catastrophic to a
person in her eighties, and these pharmaceutically-induced spills
were unacceptable. We decided, as a family, to see if an alkalizing
diet could lower her blood pressure just as effectively as the
meds, but without the miserable side effects. She took to it as
decisively as Nancy and I had, doing away with meats and dairy
in favor of juiced organic greens. With a regimen of concoctions
made from wheatgrass, cucumbers, garlic, ginger, and—integral
for its ability to fight blood pressure—hearty helpings of celery,
her systolic in now a healthy 130 over a just-as-robust diastolic
of 80. This, I should note, is without any sort of medication, and
without the accompanying dizzy spells.

As if the healing my family enjoyed hadn't been blessing
enough, fate smiled upon me one again as I'd heard word that an
old convenience store property was available for sale. I bought
it right up and established Marra's Market, a place where all-
organic, alkalizing foods are readily available for purchase for
those on their own wellness journeys. It's here that I offer what
I call the Juice of Life—100% organic vegetables run through a
juicer, just as I had done for myself, to maximize nutritional value
while doing away with the pulp that strains our systems.

I realize that my juicing and adopting an alkalizing lifestyle suggests that I might have taken a gamble, eschewing conventional medicine in favor of my two-pronged assault on acidosis. But that gamble paid off. Others, as we have seen, made similar wagers on the power of leafy greens and stress relief, and they were not let down. But should we put such measures off until we find ourselves in mortal danger? **No healthy person, for example, willfully undergoes chemo in an attempt to get even healthier. Such a thing is a last resort, a means of** *attacking disease.* **My approach, on the other hand,** *promotes well-being;* **it's a journey towards a positive end, not merely an evasion of a negative end.** It might behoove anyone, regardless of how fit he might already be, to partake in an alkalizing lifestyle. It might be the thing that staves off an otherwise impending illness. It's almost certain to shave inches off the waist. And it's virtually guaranteed not to run up your deductible. With little to lose and so much to gain, the lifestyle I'm proposing might do wonders for you.

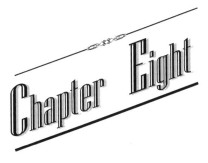

Chapter Eight

It's all because of what we eat.

LET'S LOOK ONCE AGAIN to that tale from the Book of Daniel, that reading I'd heard in Mass that seemed so tailor-made for my ears. King Nebuchadnezzar, if you'll recall, insisted that those in his service sup upon the same extravagances as he. Wise Daniel declined, opting instead for a simple diet of vegetables and water. Just like my own limited menu, Daniel's was a diet of exclusion—of doing away with the poisons.

Note too that there is no mention in the scripture of Daniel having received a dire prognosis from his oncologist. This might at first sound glib, but one must presume that if at any point Daniel had to reckon with cancer, this certainly would have been noteworthy enough to merit inclusion in the Good Book. That nothing of the sort is described would seem to imply that cancer was not an issue with which the prophet had to contend. He did not resort to what we today would call an alkalizing diet in order to beat back disease, but rather, to maintain good health. To make the point a bit differently: I could easily eat my way back into the doctor's office. I'd just have to revisit the red meats, pastas, and wines I'd indulged in before, and surely the resulting acidosis would once again prime my body for another disastrous illness. I've said it before, but it's well worth repeating; an organic, vegan diet and the elimination of stress are the keys to not merely escaping disease, but to preserving wellness.

If you've never had a horrific health scare like mine, God bless you. You can keep pressing your luck with meats and cheeses and hope that they never catch up with you—or you can take the prophet's advice, confident that spinach salads and similar green fare will stave off acidosis and keep myriad ailments at bay. In my case, it took the threat of death to whip my dietary habits into shape. Let mine be a lesson for you, too, so that you might live long, fully, and well.

So why must the Daniel diet be one of exclusion? I'd made mention above that he sought to eliminate the poisons—and that

word was no hyperbole. We in the 21ˢᵗ century are only beginning to understand the correlations between traditional American food items and different kinds of illness. The kingly court of
old Babylon must have thought it absurd for a man to turn down
the succulent meats at his disposal. But that was no mere leg of
lamb on which Daniel passed. What he was turning down, as
dieticians today know, was a bevy of health complications associ-
ated with the consumption of animal proteins and fats. Red meats
in particular are notoriously high in saturated fat. This elevates
the LDL cholesterol that puts a person at grave risk of cardiovascular disease. But it's not just your heart that's in danger; a
whole host of studies have concluded that the link between a diet
of animal proteins and cancer is very probable, and in the specific case of Colorectal Cancer, undeniable. It should be telling
that those organizations that warn against the dangers of meat
consumption include the National Institutes of Health and the
American Cancer Society. But who sinks fortunes into promoting
the supposed health benefits of beef and the like? It's none other
than the American Meat Institute, an empire which would lose a
king's ransom if folks cut meats from their diets.

Efforts in the media to describe milk and other dairy
products as essential to a healthy diet might sound a bit more
convincing. But consider that the United States Department of
Agriculture—the people who gave us that handy-dandy food
pyramid and implore us to drink three glasses of milk per day—
have, on their panel of so-called "experts," a number of dairy
industry insiders. This would seem to be yet another instance of
the almighty dollar trumping any genuine concerns for the health
of the public. Yes, there are qualified critics of dairy, and yes,
they're up in arms; sadly, they don't appear in advertisements
left and right wearing white liquid moustaches. If these dairy
detractors had better funded ad campaigns, more of us might
know, for example, that the calcium ingested from dairy foods

does nothing to ward off osteoporosis; in fact, it's in places like Asia and Africa, where dairy consumption is a rarity, that we find the fewest cases of bone deterioration. What's more, like meat, dairy is full of—you guessed it—animal proteins and saturated fats. These, as you'll recall, can lead to heart disease; counter intuitively, milk proteins also actually *contribute* to bone loss. But if enfeebled skeletal and cardiovascular systems aren't enough to scare you, consider this: regular consumption of dairy can elevate a person's insulin-like growth factor-1, or IFG-1. We know milk has vitamin D, but why don't dairy commercials boast of this other powerful element? It's very likely because IFG-1 is a known cancer-causing agent. Seems like a common thread here, doesn't it?

Previous chapters went on at length about the need for vegetables that are exclusively organic; anything less is virtually guaranteed to be ripe with chemical pesticides, fertilizers, and— the name alone is frightening enough—genetically modified organisms. Processed and enriched foods contain all of that and much, much worse. Recall the troubles I'd had with that popular breakfast cereal and its nebulous ingredients. There was a time when the term "cereal" meant just that; grain from the harvest and nothing more. Today, the average box of cereal can contain traces of as many as seventy different kinds of synthetic pesticides. But most cereals, at least, contain some semblance of what was once a natural wheat ingredient, albeit in mangled and toxic form. So many other processed foods seem more the product of Frankenstein's laboratory than any legitimate chef's kitchen. In the 20th century, we were told of the wonders of chemical preservatives, seemingly wondrous formulas that kept our foods from rotting. Chief among these are phosphate additives; they might keep a slice of processed cheese-food looking young, but they actually cause accelerated, premature aging in humans. In addition, phosphates have been shown to inhibit kidney function

and, like so many other foods on our list, contribute to bone loss.
Consuming this nefarious additive is enough to ensure that you
won't simply look old before your time; you'll feel it, too. But
phosphates are hardly the end of our troubles. It's next to im-
possible to find a product on the supermarket shelf that doesn't
contain enriched flour, white sugar, or trans fats. These and other
"refined" ingredients have been shown to cause inflammation of
the tissue. Chronic inflammation is a known culprit behind such
conditions as respiratory failure, cardiovascular disease, neuro-
logical disorders such as dementia, and of course, my old nemesis
cancer. There goes that common thread popping up once again.

When Daniel insisted that his sole beverage would be water,
the context of the ancient Mediterranean world would imply
that he was in fact saying no to wine. While the fact that alcohol
is a thing to be avoided should be obvious enough, I would be
remiss not to say a few words on the subject. Many of us think
that so long as we can evade a drunk driving charge, and at
least not drink our livers rotten, we're in the clear. Vehicular
homicide and cirrhosis should be enough to give a person pause
under any circumstances, but these are hardly the only risks we
take when we overindulge. Drinking to excess can have a hugely
negative impact on the makeup of our blood. It leeches the
system of vitamin B, deforming our red blood cells and causing
anemia. These warped cells are then that much more likely to
clump together into clots, which can result in strokes and heart
attacks. And for those readers anxious for that common thread
to once again rear its head: as the body digests alcohol, our
systems convert the stuff into acetaldehyde. This is among the
most powerful carcinogens known to man. It might take us out
quickly, or it might spend decades teasing us torturously; to stave
off acidosis and so much more, alcohol is a thing to steer clear of.

I feel it's important to bring up one more offender when it
comes to detrimental items we put into our body: Aspartame,

or more specifically, ALL artificial sweeteners in existence today. Even Stevia, due to the way it's manufactured and processed, can be highly dangerous and even toxic to the digestive system!

The biggest offender of artificial sweeteners, and it should go without saying, is high fructose corn syrup. There have been numerous studies about the dangers of ingesting high fructose corn syrup and its ill effects, but I think it's important to mention that it contributes to fat deposits in the liver, leads to plaque buildup and narrowing of blood vessels, and makes us highly susceptible to diseases like diabetes, obesity, and arguably…cancer.

How can high fructose corn syrup be so terrible for our bodies, you ask? Well, some basic biochemistry can help you understand its negative effects more clearly. See, regular cane sugar (i.e., sucrose) is made of two sugar molecules, fructose and glucose, that are bound pretty close together and in an even amount of molecules. High fructose corn syrup is extracted from sucrose using a chemical enzymatic process that makes the ratio of fructose and glucose uneven, with there being more fructose than glucose in an unbound form. The reason why this is significant is because when the enzymes inside your digestive tract breaks down the high fructose corn syrup, it requires much more energy than it would normally need for breaking down sucrose. The depletion of energy actually ends up weakening your intestinal lining that is responsible for keeping bacteria and food from leaking across the intestinal membrane, causing widespread inflammation in your body. High fructose literally punches holes in the intestinal lining, which allows all the awful by products of toxic gut bacteria and partially digested food proteins to enter the bloodstream unchecked.

If this wasn't bad enough, the fructose molecules are rapidly absorbed into your bloodstream and go straight to your liver. This is why high fructose corn syrup is a major cause of liver damage and contributes to the diseases like diabetes and obesity. In fact, the metabolic disturbances are so disruptive to your internal homeostasis that cancer can creep right into your life, and with enough stress to propel cancer to its more serious stages, will eventually cause your life to be in jeopardy.

And to think, it's all because of what we eat.

Chapter Nine

OKAY, SO I'VE DISCUSSED WHAT WE CAN'T EAT, but what about the food that is acceptable for consumption? And how exactly should a healthy diet compliment your attempt to lead a stress free life? I feel it's important to recap everything so far and provide you with some lists to live by. Let's pull this all together so you can be on your way to living a cancer free life.

The very first step is to check your pH level. How acidic are you? It's important to know exactly what level of acidity you are dealing with before trying to maintain a healthy pH balance in your bloodstream. You can check your pH levels easily at home with paper pH strips. I recommend using pH strips, as you can get them at most pharmacies, but if you want something a little more hi-tech, you can always opt for a pH electron meter. You might have to order this online or purchase it from a health catalogue though.

With pH strips, you test the pH of your saliva or urine, though I would recommend testing only your urine. It is more consistent in its results than saliva and also changes in response to what you eat. When you test your pH, the ideal blood pH you are looking for is 7.365. Anything below 7 is considered acidic and anything above it is considered basic, or alkaline. So having a very mildly basic blood pH is the key.

NEXT, IN ORDER TO HELP BOTH ACHIEVE AND MAINTAIN THE PROPER PH BALANCE, THE FOLLOWING ITEMS SHOULD BE CONSIDERED:

1. **VEGETABLES/RAW FOODS:** This should be the focus of your diet. Review the list I provided in Chapter Six, go online for more extensive options to consider, and remember above all, **all your vegetable choices must be organic!**

2. **GRASSES:** These are incredibly nutrient-dense and full of Chlorophyll, which is what gives grass its regenerative effect. This creates a similar effect on a molecular and cellular level in your body.

3. **LOW-CARBOHYDRATE VEGETABLES:** You can eat high-carbohydrate vegetables but only in moderation. The core and focus of your vegetable consumption must be low-carbohydrate veggies, including fresh legumes, fresh grains, and sprouts.

4. **SOY (NOT GENETICALLY MODIFIED):** This is a great source of protein and also has a huge source of wonderful nutrients for your body.

5. **FRESH FISH:** If you decide to flavor your meal selections with fish, do so sparingly, as fish can create acidity in the bloodstream. But fish is also a fantastic source of omega-3 oils and proteins. Be sure the fish is fresh and comes from unpolluted water if you decide to include it in your meals.

6. **SPROUTS:** I believe these are the very best foods you can eat. Sprouts are living plant foods packed with enzymes, complete proteins, minerals, and vitamins. Some examples of great sprouts to digest include green lentil sprouts, sesame sprouts, sunflower sprouts, chickpea sprouts, and wheat sprouts. This list is by no means exhaustive; there are plenty of sprouts in the world to choose from, so I encourage you to do some exploration and taste testing to find out what sprouts appeal the most to you.

7. **HERBS AND SPICES:** These are useful to keeping things tasting great for you. They also can help with building up your immune system. Be sure they are fresh and you should have no problem including herbs and spices into your diet.

8. **TOMATO AND AVOCADO:** When these are eaten raw, they have an alkalizing effect in the body. Both are a great source of protein as well and have excellent potassium levels, which means you can skip eating sugary bananas for your potassium needs!

THE ABOVE LIST SHOULD BE COMPLIMENTED WITH APPROPRIATE DRINKS. I RECOMMEND THE FOLLOWING:

1. **WATER:** alkaline water that is fresh and pure, about one gallon every day. Make sure the water you drink is not direct from your tap or in bottles you buy at the store. Your water needs to be filtered correctly through distillation, which can be achieved with simple filters you can buy anywhere.

2. **JUICE:** Vegetable juices only, particularly green vegetables and grasses. Juicing is my main weapon against imbalance of pH in my blood. It should be yours too.

While eating right and ingesting proper liquids is both important and essential in maintaining proper pH balance in your bloodstream, you can still do more for yourself to insure that you're getting an added boost of protection against the harmful chemicals and pollutants your bodies are subjected to every single day. I'm talking about dietary supplements, which will compliment your overall quest for optimal health. Supplements aren't intended to be used in place of eating but rather to compliment your diets, and they normally provide huge sums of vitamins, minerals, herbs, amino acids and more. Colloidal supplements (i.e., liquid supplements) are particularly useful, as they pass through membranes inside the body very easily. No energy gets wasted when ingesting them. Below is a small but comprehensive list of supplements to consider:

1. **CONCENTRATED GREEN POWDER**
2. **ESSENTIAL FATTY ACIDS**
3. **MULTIVITAMINS**
4. **MULTI-MINERAL FORMULA WITH CELL SALTS**
5. **PH DROPS**
6. **CHLOROPHYLL**
7. **PINE BARK EXTRACT.**
8. **ENZYMES* (SEE NEXT SECTION)**

I would be remiss if I didn't let you know that there are hundreds, if not thousands, of supplements out there on the market today. Be sure to research any supplements that interest you, and also check to see if they've been dutifully tested, as some supplements could end up being dangerous to you instead of helpful.

One supplement that deserves attention is enzymes. If you think about it, enzymes can be considered the foundation for all cell regeneration, as they play the vital role in the transformation of undigested food into nutrients that ourcells can absorb and use in daily body processes.

THERE ARE THREE CATEGORIES OF ENZYMES, OF WHICH THOUSANDS OF ENZYMES CAN BE GROUPED INTO:

DIGESTIVE ENZYMES: These are utilized by the digestive system to break down food. Examples of digestive enzymes include protease, amylase, and lipase.

METABOLIC ENZYMES: These are found in every cell, tissue, and organ in our bodies. They enhance the life of every cell.

FOOD ENZYMES: These usually come from raw, uncooked foods. Fresh produce contains food enzymes too.

After you've established a food diet that is complimented with nutritious drinks and supplements, what now? Remember, eating and drinking right is essential to living a healthy life, but it's not enough to stop cancer in its tracks. You must make sure to eliminate stress in your life. Just as Dr. Coldwell believes, I am just as convicted about stress being the leading source and cause for cancer to appear in our lives. Of course there are exceptions to this, such as if you were exposed to radiation, poisoning, or physical trauma that induces cancer in some form. But without a doubt, physical, emotional, and mental stress aggravate what is happening on our bodies. Specifically the pH levels getting out of whack and creating acidity that is harmful to our wellbeing. I've discussed this in Chapter Five but it's worth mentioning again-getting rid of all distress in your life equals a much higher chance at becoming cancer free.

The final part of the equation for beating cancer and living healthy overall is to have the proper motivation. For me, it's my faith. I am firmly convinced that this is the only kind of motivation that works, but regardless of what motivates you, there has to be a sense of spirituality grounded into your actions when confronting something so deadly as a disease or improper pH balance in your blood. To have the right motivation means you will always be focused and determined in making sure you are never going down the incorrect path when it comes to safely eating and living. I recommend taking the time in your day or week or month to do a checklist of the things that are working for you and the things that are holding you back. It's important to define your goals in life: What do you want to achieve before you die? What are you trying to accomplish or create or write or play or read or see or do? I also believe that you should have some sense of the world around you and the world you can't see around us all; I'm talking about a spiritual awareness. Even if you are an atheist or don't believe in God, you can still adhere to the idea that this life has to have more meaning than just living and dying. If you can establish that there is something more to existence, then imagine how powerful a motivational tool this can be for you to try and search and discover another reason to live each day to the fullest? If you do believe in God, then I don't need to tell you how important it is to live your life in the best way possible, respecting the Golden Rule in dealing with others, and subscribing to modesty and moderation in all things. I believe this is the perfect path to being stress free, as well as setting up the backdrop to taking on the difficult but necessary challenge of changing your lifestyle and eating habits to achieve a perfect pH balance in every meal selection.

EATING RIGHT

+

DRINKING RIGHT

+

ELIMINATION OF STRESS

+

MOTIVATION

=

CANCER FREE!!!

Conclusion

AS I THINK ABOUT MY LIFE and how I have overcome cancer, I am hopeful that my body will continue to respond to the new lifestyle choices I've made and keep me cancer free. But what if it does come back? I am always mindful of what cancer actually is, and you should be too.

We can define it a number of ways, but probably the best way to think about cancer is that it's a collection of dead cells and mutated or damaged cells in our bodies. Our immune system is set up to normally eliminate the accumulation of these used up cells. But for whatever reason, whether it's from acidosis, toxins, or unnatural events like radiation exposure, if these cells manage to build up too much in our systems, the cells have a chance to become abnormal and start dividing without any control function in place. These cells begin to invade tissues and other parts of the body. The cells themselves that should die or be cleaned up as part of the daily cellular maintenance keep splitting and growing and eventually can form a mass of tissue we all know as a tumor. So then, if we eat poorly, are constantly stressed out, and ingest fluids that are full of toxins and junk our body doesn't need, we lower our immune system's ability to maintain cellular reproduction and cleanup, thus opening the door to cancer and actually a host of other diseases.

In the spirit of humility, I must once again remind everyone that this my aforementioned description of cancer and what happens is purely based on my experience with it and what I've read regarding treatment of the disease. However, I am firm in my thoughts about what to do when cancer shows up and how to prevent cancer from ever showing up in my life again. I hope with this minuscule description of cancer that I've just provided you can see how important it is to have a relatively stress free life that is full of good eatin' and good livin'! And don't get me wrong-I'm not suggesting you live like an ascetic monk and practice absolute abstinence from pleasurable sweets or walking away from situations that will require stress to overcome them. I believe that this blueprint for your life that I've set out is not an ideal way to live on a permanent basis. I want everyone to consider that when I received the terrible news from my doctor that I had cancer, I found a way to defeat it by practicing everything in this book. And I've seen how the formula I've provided in this book of stress elimination plus eating and drinking right plus being motivated spiritually work just the same way for my wife and mother-in-law as it did for me. It's something you must do 100% and never waiver even once, but the key is that you **practice this lifestyle of positivity only when you begin to experience cancer or other diseases and continue to live in a health-conscious way until you are free and in the clear of your malady.** Of course I strongly encourage you to live in the manner I've suggested in this book *all the time*, but I realize that most of us might not be able to make such a huge lifestyle change that easily. And that's okay.

> PRACTICE THIS LIFESTYLE OF POSITIVITY ONLY WHEN YOU BEGIN TO EXPERIENCE CANCER OR OTHER DISEASES AND CONTINUE TO LIVE IN A HEALTH-CONSCIOUS WAY UNTIL YOU ARE FREE AND IN THE CLEAR OF YOUR MALADY.

Think about this just for a moment: We now live in an age where it's possible to indulge in just about anything on a massive level. There are fast food restaurants on every corner of every city in America. Grocery stores carry products loaded with harmful chemicals that slowly over time eradicate our insides. We have television and online video aggregates like YouTube constantly full of stressful news and images. I mean, you can go on YouTube right now and watch actual death over and over again, as much as you want to indulge in the macabre. When I think about Daniel and when he lived, there was absolutely nothing like this in existence. It was easier to ingest foods that were natural and healthy. Likewise, there was stress in the world, but it was limited to what a person mostly heard, unless they lived in an area plagued by war or chose to insert themselves in stressful situations. And everyone back then seemed to have a sense of the spiritual world. It was easier to accept God and the realm of the invisible, as few didn't bow down at the altar of technology and humanism. It's no wonder to me that in the Bible, there's no mention of cancer. I haven't read or seen any historical documents from Biblical times that describe anything even close to cancer. I'm not saying it didn't exist back then, but then again, I wouldn't be surprised if it didn't either. I imagine that the answer to healthy living must be somewhere in the fact that eating right, eliminating stress from life, and being motivated either spiritually or on any kind of purposeful level is truly the way to be permanently healthy and live a long-lasting and fulfilling life. So it's my ardent wish for all of you who took the time to read about my ordeal with cancer and how I beat it to stop, even for a moment, and consider that what I'm proposing can only help you and not hurt you. I feel great, I live great, and I believe in the Great Almighty God, and will continue to act and feel this way forever.

"*It should be forbidden and severely punished to remove cancer by cutting, burning, cautery, and other fiendish tortures. It is from nature that the disease comes, and from nature comes the cure, not from physicians.*"

PARACELSUS (1493-1541 AD)

78

HIGHEST ALKALINE	ALKALINE	LOWEST ALKALINE
STEVIA	MAPLE SYRUP RICE SYRUP	RAW SUGAR RAW HONEY
LEMONS LIMES WATERMELON GRAPEFRUIT MANGOES PAPAYAS	DRIED FRUIT MELONS GRAPES KIWI BERRIES APPLES, PEARS	BANANAS CHERRIES PINEAPPLE ORANGES PEACHES
ASPARAGUS BROCCOLI ONIONS VEGETABLE JUICES RAW SPINACH PARSLEY LENTILS GARLIC	CARROTS GREEN BEANS CELERY LETTUCE ZUCCHINI BEETS SWEET POTATO CAROB	AVOCADOS MUSHROOMS CORN CABBAGE PEAS POTATO SKINS OLIVES SOYBEANS TOFU
	ALMONDS	CHESTNUTS
OLIVE OIL	FLAX SEED OIL	CANOLA OIL
		AMARANTH MILLET WILD RICE QUINOA
	BREAST MILK ALMOND MILK	GOAT MILK SOY MILK GOAT CHEESE SOY CHEESE
MINERAL WATER LEMON WATER HERB TEAS	GREEN TEA KAMBUCHA SPRING WATER	GINGER TEA
BAKING SODA SEA SALT CHLORELLA KELP	SPICES CLOVER MINT PARSNIP	GRAIN COFFEE SPROUTS CURRANT

ALKALIZING

ALKALIZING MINERALS

CALCIUM: PH 12
CESIUM: PH 14
MAGNESIUM: PH 9
POTASSIUM: PH 14
SODIUM: PH 14

FOODS

ALKALINE AND ACID FOOD CHART

FOOD CATEGORY	LOWEST ACID	ACID	MOST ACID
SWEETENERS	MOLASSES PROCESSED HONEY	SUGAR	ALL ARTIFICIAL SWEETNERS
FRUITS	DATES BLUEBERRIES CRANBERRIES PLUMS PROCESSED FRUIT COCONUT	POMEGRANATE CANNED FRUIT SOUR CHERRIES RHUBARB	BLACKBERRIES CRANBERRIES PRUNES
VEGETABLES BEANS LEGUMES	SESAME SEEDS FAVA BEANS STRING BEANS KIDNEY BEANS COOKED SPINACH BLACK-EYED PEAS	PINTO BEANS NAVY BEANS POTATOES CHICK PEA	SOYBEAN CHOCOLATE PICKLED- VEGETABLES
NUTS SEEDS	PUMPKIN SEEDS SUNFLOWER SEEDS	CASHEWS PECANS PISTACHIOS	PEANUTS WALNUTS
OILS	CORN OIL	SUNFLOWER OIL	SESAME OIL
CEREALS GRAINS	BROWN RICE SPELT SPROUTED WHOLE- WHEAT BREAD	WHITE RICE CORNMEAL BUCKWHEAT OATS & RYE	WHEAT WHITE FLOUR PASTRIES PASTA
MEATS	VENISON COLD WATER FISH	TURKEY LAMB CHICKEN	BEEF PORK SHELLFISH
EGGS DAIRY	EGGS BUTTER YOGURT BUTTERMILK	COTTAGE CHEESE HARD CHEESE RAW MILK RICE MILK	CUSTARD ICE CREAM MILK CHEESE
BEVERAGES	TEA DISTILLED WATER RED WINE	COCOA COFFEE WHITE WINE	BEER LIQUOR SOFT DRINKS
MISC	MARGARINE LARD MSG	MUSTARD JELLIES AND JAMS KETCHUP MAYONNAISE	COCOA CANDY CONFECTIONERY PRESERVATIVES

IN ORDER TO LIVE HEALTHY AND ENCOURAGE YOUR BODY TO STAY FREE OF DISEASES LIKE CANCER, HERE ARE SOME RECIPES STRAIGHT FROM MY KITCHEN. USE THEM AND I GUARANTEE YOU WILL BE ON YOUR WAY TO FEELING WONDERFUL EACH AND EVERY DAY OF YOUR LIFE!

*Note: For all recipes, I recommend ALL ORGANIC INGREDIENTS ONLY.

Recipes

DIRECTIONS:

1. Wash all organic vegetables thoroughly.

2. Trim and cut the organic vegetables to fit into the juicer's opening.

3. Feed the wheat grass first, a little at a time, followed by all the organic leafy greens with a few organic carrots to push them through.

4. Feed the balance of the vegetables finishing with the rest of the organic carrots.

5. All organic vegetables and quantities can be varied according to taste and benefit or by what is available to juice.

6. A dash or three of cayenne pepper can be added for an anti-inflammatory kick!

ENJOY YOUR PURE, NUTRIENT FILLED RAW FOOD!

*IF YOU ARE CURIOUS ABOUT WHAT KIND OF JUICER TO USE, I RECOMMEND THE OMEGA 8004 SLOW COLD PRESSED MASTICATING JUICER, OR SOMETHING EQUAL.

MY DAILY JUICE OF LIFE

I JUICE WITH THE FOLLOWING ALL ORGANIC
VEGETABLES AT LEAST 1-2 TIMES DAILY,
TYPICALLY FOR BREAKFAST AND LUNCH.

1 CUCUMBER

1 LB. CELERY

½ LB. CARROTS

1 APPLE

1-2 PCS. OF KALE

1-2 HANDFULS OF SPINACH

SLICE OF GINGER
(FOR SPICE)

½ SM. JUICING BEET

¼ - ½ LEMON

2 OZ. WHEAT GRASS

DIRECTIONS:

1. Cook the quinoa pasta according to the directions on the box and set aside. Do not over cook.

2. Start by stir-frying the broccoli on high heat for 5 minutes.

3. Add oil as needed or to prevent vegetables from sticking.

4. Keep on high heat and add quinoa pasta until slightly browned.

5. Reduce to medium heat and add cayenne and sea salt for taste.

**8 OZ. QUINOA
PENNE PASTA**
(COOKED AL-DENTE)

4 TO 6 CROWNS BROCCOLI
CUT BITE SIZE FOR FORK
TENDER CRISPNESS

4-6 CLOVES OF GARLIC

**¼ - ½ CUP OF
EXTRA VIRGIN
OLIVE OIL**

CAYENNE PEPPER

DIRECTIONS:

1. Cook your choice of Quinoa noodle or grain per the instruction on the box and set aside.

2. Boil water and add BETTER THAN BOUILLON "NO CHICKEN BASE".

3. Add two small sweet onions pureed in a food processor until smooth.

4. Add carrots to mixture and olive oil.

5. Bring to a boil until the carrots are fork tender then shut off the pot.

6. Add rinsed beans and fresh spinach while stirring and let sit until ready to be served.

7. Bring to a simmer and serve immediately over quinoa noodle.

8. Add sea salt to taste.

NOTE

DO NOT BOIL SPINACH.
NUTRITIONAL VALUE WILL BE LOST AND
ACIDITY WILL OCCUR.

ITALIAN VEGAN WEDDING SOUP

8 OZ. COOKED ORGANIC QUINOA PASTA SHELLS OR ELBOWS OR QUINOA GRAIN

2 SMALL ONIONS

4-5 HANDFULS OF FRESH SPINACH

2 - 15 OZ. CANS OF CANNELLINI BEANS
(DRAINED AND RINSED)

1 - 15 OZ. CAN OF GREAT NORTHERN OR PINTO BEANS
(DRAINED AND RINSED)

1 CUP OF DICED CARROTS

2 QUARTS OF WATER

¼ CUP EXTRA VRGIN OLIVE OIL

4-5 TEASPOONS OF BETTER THAN BOUILLON
«NO CHICKEN BASE» BRAND OR ANY OTHER ORGANIC VEGETABLE BASE

DIRECTIONS:

1. Puree all 4 cans of tomatoes and set aside.

2. Sautee onions in olive oil until onions are translucent but not brown.

3. Add diced cloves of garlic and quickly fry with already translucent onion, but do not brown the garlic all the way.

4. Add pureed tomatoes with juice to the onions and garlic and cook for 10-15 minutes on medium heat.

5. Add basil if you prefer a heavier tasting marinara sauce.

6. If tomato taste is too strong or acidic, bring the pot to boil and add 1/8 teaspoon of baking soda to reduce acidity until the acid taste is gone.

ALTERNATIVE

ADD TO YOUR LIKING ORGANIC HONEY, ONE TEASPOON AT A TIME, TO OFF-SET ACID THAT MAY OCCUR AFTER COOKING TOMATOES.

3 - 28 OZ. ORGANIC WHOLE TOMATOES PACKED IN ITS OWN JUICE
(WOODSTOCK OR MUIR GLEN)

1 – 28 OZ. TOMATO SAUCE
(WOODSTOCK OR MUIR GLEN)

¼ CUP EXTRA VIRGIN OLIVE OIL

1 MEDIUM SIZED ONION DICED

4 DICED CLOVES OF GARLIC

SALT AND PEPPER TO TASTE

¼ TEASPOON OF BASIL
(OPTIONAL)

½ - 1 LB. ORGANIC QUINOA PASTA
OR ANY ORGANIC PASTA OF YOUR CHOICE
COOKED AL-DENTE

DIRECTIONS:

1. Cook wild rice or quinoa according to directions, then drain and set aside.

2. Sauté bite size broccoli by adding olive oil to pureed zucchini and celery.

3. Puree in processor 6 stalks of celery and two medium size zucchini.

4. Pour in large boiling pot of water.

5. Add vegetable base and bring to full boil after adding remaining celery until broccoli is fork tender and the fresh beans begin to soften.

6. Next add canned or defrosted lima beans with Italian seasoning, stirring constantly.

7. Add remaining cubed zucchini and diced celery and mix again

8. Next add minced garlic and stir.

9. Add sea salt and cayenne pepper for taste.

10. Cook on low heat for the next 10 minutes and serve hot over long grain wild rice or quinoa pasta.

8 OZ. OF LONG GRAIN WILD RICE
OR QUINOA ELBOWS OR SHELLS

2 QUARTS OF WATER

4-5 TEASPOONS OF BETTER THAN BOUILLON
«NO CHICKEN BASE» BRAND
OR ANY OTHER ORGANIC VEGETABLE BASE

3 CLOVES GARLIC DICED

**4-6 CROWNS OF BROCCOLI FLORETS
CUT IN BITE SIZE**

**2 HANDFULS OF FRESH SNIPPED AND
WASHED FRESH GREEN BEANS CUT IN HALF**
OR 2 CANS OF ORGANIC CANNED GREEN BEANS

4 MEDIUM SIZE ZUCCHINI CUBED

1 PACKAGE OF FROZEN LIMA BEANS
OR 1 SMALL 8 OZ. CAN OF LIMA BEANS

**12 STALKS OF WASHED ORGANIC
CELERY DICED**

**1 TABLESPOON OF ORGANIC
ITALIAN SEASONING**

SEA SALT AND CAYENNE PEPPER TO TASTE

DIRECTIONS:

1. Heat olive oil in a large boiling pot.

2. Purée onion and zucchini in processor and mix together, then place in pot.

3. Add carrots and celery and sauté over low heat until fork tender.

4. Add water and vegetable base while stirring and bring to a full boil.

5. Reduce heat and carefully stir in rinsed beans.

6. Add fresh minced garlic.

7. Add honey to reduce acidity one spoonful at a time.

8. Add water, if necessary, for consistency of soup.

9. Taste and season with sea salt and pepper as necessary.

10. Shut off heat and serve hot over quinoa noodles.

NOTE

ADD HONEY IF ACIDITY AND OR BITTERNESS OCCUR
TO OFFSET ACID FROM TOMATOES.
SERVE WITH GREEN SALAD.
GOES GREAT WITH RED ORGANIC WINE!

PASTA E FAGIOLI SOUP

HIGH IN PROTEIN AND FIBER

8 OZ. BOX OF QUINOA ELBOWS OR SHELLS
(COOKED ACCORDING TO DIRECTIONS)

1- 28 OZ. CAN OF TOMATO PURÉE

1- 15 OZ. CAN OF CANNELLINI BEANS

1- 15 OZ. CAN OF RED OR PINTO BEANS

1- 15 OZ. CAN OF SMALL GREAT NORTHERN BEANS

2 QUARTS OF WATER

6 CLOVES OF MINCED GARLIC

½ CUP OLIVE OIL

2 CUPS OF DICED CELERY

2 CUPS OF DICED CARROTS

2 LARGE ZUCCHIN

1 LARGE ONION

2 CUPS CHOPPED CELERY

2 CUPS CHOPPED CARROTS

4-5 TEASPOONS OF BETTER THAN BOUILLON
«NO CHICKEN BASE» BRAND
OR ANY OTHER ORGANIC VEGETABLE BASE

5 TABLESPOONS OF HONEY AS NECESSARY

DIRECTIONS:

1. Rinse beans with cold water and drain well. Use a large mixing bowl to do this.

2. Add the onion, garlic, and red pepper with half of the dressing and toss lightly using a large spoon.

3. Add the chopped parsley and the remaining dressing. Mix well.

4. Store in a covered container and refrigerate for future use.

NOTE

YOU MAY ADD MORE SALT AND/OR VINEGAR FOR TASTE. HOWEVER, IF YOU CHOOSE TO USE THE INGREDIENTS LISTED FOR THE DRESSING, MAKE SURE TO SHAKE THE INGREDIENTS TOGETHER IN A SHAKER BEFORE APPLYING TO THE SALAD.

ITALIAN ORGANIC BEAN SALAD

1 - 15 OZ. CAN BLACK BEANS

1 - 15 OZ. CAN GARBANZO BEANS

1 - 15 OZ. CAN BLACK-EYED PEAS

1 - 15 OZ. CAN PINTO BEANS

1 - 15 OZ. CAN WHOLE KERNEL CORN

1 - 15 OZ. CAN NAVY OR CANNELLINI BEANS

2 TABLESPOONS MINCED FRESH GARLIC

1 DICED LARGE RED BELL PEPPER

1 SCANT CUP CHOPPED RED ONION

1 CUP (PACKED) CHOPPED FRESH PARSLEY
(CUT OFF LARGE STEMS AND USE LEAVES ONLY)

FOR THE DRESSING

¼ CUP WHITE BALSAMIC VINEGAR

½ CUP CANOLA OIL

2 TEASPOONS SEA SALT

¼ TEASPOON BLACK PEPPER

¼ TEASPOON STEVIA

DIRECTIONS:

1. Heat in a large frying pan or electric skillet organic olive oil with 4 to 6 minced garlic cloves.

2. Start by stir-frying the broccoli first on high heat for 5 minutes.

3. Add oil as needed or to stop vegetables from sticking.

4. Reduce to medium heat and add remainder of vegetables until fork tender crispness.

5. Keep on medium heat and add more garlic, organic pepper, and sea salt for taste.

6. Serve over long grain wild rice, quinoa grain, or any quinoa pasta of your choice.

7. Stir-fry sauce optional on the side.

RECOMMENDED
TAMARI ORGANIC SOY OR TERIYAKI SAUCE FOR ADDED FLAVOR.

2 CUPS LONG GRAIN WILD RICE OR QUINOA GRAIN
(COOKED AL-DENTE)

10 SMALL BRUSSEL SPROUTS SLICED IN HALF

2 BUNCHES OF ASPARAGUS
(HEADS ARE PREFERABLE)

2 SMALL ZUCCHINI SLICED OR CUBED FOR BITE SIZE

6 TO 8 CROWNS OF BROCCOLI, CUT BITE SIZE FOR FORK TENDER CRISPNESS

¼ - ½ CUP OF EXTRA VIRGIN OLIVE OIL

DIRECTIONS:

1. Warm a skillet over medium heat. Add the pine nuts to the skillet. Stir them continuously until they are toasted golden brown. Remove from heat.

2. Add toasted pine nuts to a food processor along with 4 cups of fresh, clean basil leaves.

3. Process the nuts and leaves together into small pieces. Scrape the sides of the processor.

4. Add 1/3 cup extra virgin olive oil along with the garlic and lemon juice.

5. Process again, scraping the sides periodically, until the mixture becomes creamy.

6. Mix in the grated cheese, adding more olive oil if desired, to create a smooth paste.

7. Add more sea salt to taste, if needed (taste your mixture first, as you may not need any if your cheese is on the salty side).

8. Make the pasta of your choice (I recommend quinoa spaghetti or linguine).

9. Cook to your desired hardness and drain well (do not rinse) and immediately mix in pesto while it's steaming hot. Coat the pasta evenly.

NOTE

PESTO CAN ALSO BE USED OVER GLUTEN FREE PIZZA SHELLS.

BASIL PESTO SAUCE

¼ CUP PINE NUTS
(⅓ CUP FOR VEGAN RECIPE)

4 CUPS FRESH BASIL LEAVES

⅓ CUP EXTRA VIRGIN OLIVE OIL

4 CLOVES ROASTED GARLIC
(OR 2 CLOVES UNROASTED)

½ FRESH LEMON, JUICED
(FOR TASTE)

½ CUP GRATED PECORINO OR PARMESAN CHEESE
(OMIT FOR VEGAN AND SUBSTITUTE
WITH ⅓ CUP GRATED RAW
CASHEWS OR ALMONDS AND
1 TSP. OF SEA SALT)

DIRECTIONS:

1. Cook quinoa according to directions and allow to fully cool.

2. Mix sesame oil and cooked quinoa thoroughly.

3. Add sesame seeds and raisins and stir together into mixture.

4. Add pistachios and soy into mixture.

5. Mix everything together and chill before serving.

6. Add sea salt to taste

2 CUPS COOKED QUINOA
(COOK UNTIL SPROUTS EMERGE
BUT NOT MUSHY)

1 CUP OF RIPE RED RAISINS

4 TABLESPOONS OF ORGANIC SOY SAUCE

½ CUP CRUSHED PISTACHIOS

1 CUP SESAME SEED OIL

2 TABLESPOONS TOASTED SESAME SEEDS
(GROUND AND SALTED IF POSSIBLE)

DIRECTIONS:

1. Rinse and strain all beans well.

2. Add all ingredients together EXCEPT avocado and salt. Stir well.

3. Add sea salt and avocado and gently toss. Serve chilled or at room temperature.

4. Serve with choice of organic tortilla chips.

5. To make spicier add a double pinch of cayenne pepper.

1 - 15 OZ. CAN WHOLE KERNEL CORN

1 - 15 OZ. CAN OF BLACK BEANS

1 - 15 OZ. CAN OF GARBANZO BEANS

1 CUP OF BALSAMIC VINEGAR

1 DICED RIPE AVOCADO

½ PINT OF CHERRY TOMATOES CUT IN HALF

1 DICED RED BELL PEPPER

SEA SALT
(RECOMMEND 1 TABLESPOON)

A PINCH OF CAYENNE PEPPER
(IF YOU WANT TO GIVE YOUR CAVIAR AN EXTRA KICK!)

MIXING DIRECTIONS NOT NECESSARY

ALL INGREDIENTS ARE OPTIONAL AND MAY BE ADDED, DELETED OR SUBSTITUTED ACCORDING TO YOUR TASTE.

1 HEAD ROMAINE LETTUCE

8 OZ. FRESH BABY SPINACH

4 CELERY STALKS

1 CUCUMBER

1-2 CARROTS

1 MEDIUM SIZE TOMATO OR A PINT OF CHERRY TOMATOES

1 GREEN AND RED PEPPERS

ONIONS

4 TABLESPOONS BALSAMIC VINEGAR

4 TABLESPOONS EXTRA VIRGIN OLIVE OIL

SEA SALT

DIRECTIONS:

1. Begin with a teaspoon of Dr. Todd's Matcha Tea (or any Matcha Tea) in a large mug and add boiling water.

2. Heat one half teaspoon of baking soda and four teaspoons of grade B organic maple syrup in a small butter warmer pot to a froth (do not overheat). Add it to the tea.

3. Add two to three scoops of hulled hemp seed (loaded with omega 3 and 6) for a nutty flavor and stir slowly.

4. Let it sit for three minutes.

ENJOY THE ALKALINITY!

DR. TODD'S MATCHA TEA
(OR ANY MATCHA TEA)

½ TEASPOON BAKING SODA

4 TEASPOONS GRADE B ORGANIC MAPLE SYRUP

2-3 SCOOPS HULLED HEMP SEED

DIRECTIONS:

1. Preheat oven to 375 degrees.

2. Slice spaghetti squash in half length wise. Make sure to use a large sharp knife.

3. Scoop out seeds and throw away.

4. Place cut side down on a rimmed cookie sheet covered in water.

5. Bake about 45-55 minutes or until fork tender.

6. Once the squash is cooked, gently spread the spaghetti toward the center going along the grain. Evenly spread the organic extra virgin olive oil on both halves.

7. Sprinkle with the sea salt and organic black pepper.

8. Place back in the oven for about 5-10 min.

9. Scoop and place in a bowl and add salt and pepper to taste.

10. Once the squash is cooked and shredded, it can be topped with a marinara sauce or pesto and toasted pine nuts or any of your favorite pasta toppings.

11. Add a little grated cheese.

1 MEDIUM SIZE SPAGHETTI SQUASH

1 TABLESPOON EXTRA VIRGIN OLIVE OIL

1/2 TEASPOON SEA SALT

1/2 TEASPOON FINE GROUND BLACK PEPPER

DIRECTIONS:

1. Cook lentils according to directions, then rinse, drain, and set aside.

2. Purée 2 small zucchini with skins, 1 apple, and 6 stalks of celery.

3. With celery and 1 large onion in processor, place in soup pot and add 4 cups of water.

4. Add remaining diced celery, diced carrots, and diced apples to puréed vegetables.

5. Add 2 tablespoons of olive oil.

6. Bring to a boil for two to three minutes.

7. Reduce to simmer while stirring.

8. Add 8 cups of water mixed with "Better than Boullion" or any organic vegetable base of your choice

9. Slowly add turmeric for light nutty flavor and desired color for soup

10. Add lentils while stirring.

11. Bring to a boil for another 2 -3 minutes, then shut off and serve.

**2 BUNCHES OF CELERY OR 12
STALKS OF CELERY, DICED**

**2 SMALL ZUCCHINI
WITH SKINS, DICED**

**3 SWEET AVERAGE SIZE RED
APPLES, CORED, PEELED AND DICED**

1 LARGE YELLOW ONION, PEELED

4 LARGE CARROTS, DICED

**2 TABLESPOONS
TURMERIC SPICE**

**2 CUPS OF RED, BLACK OR GREEN
LENTILS**

**4-5 TEASPOONS OF BETTER
THAN BOUILLON
"NO CHICKEN BASE" BRAND**
OR ANY OTHER ORGANIC VEGETABLE BASE

ACKNOWLEDGMENTS

BESIDES GOD, WHO WAS MERCIFUL TO ME AND GAVE ME THE WISDOM AND STRENGTH TO FIGHT MY GRIM DIAGNOSIS, MY NEXT BIGGEST THANK YOU BELONGS TO MY INCREDIBLE WIFE NANCY. WITHOUT HER I COULDN'T HAVE BEATEN CANCER; FROM HER ENDLESS PRAYERS TO ALWAYS BEING IN THE KITCHEN, WHIPPING UP MY CURING FOODS, SHE WAS WITH ME EVERY DISCIPLINED STEP OF THE WAY. I ALSO WANT TO THANK DR. TODD PESEK, MY HOLISTIC DOCTOR, WHO TOLD ME I WAS GOING TO BEAT MY CANCER, KEPT HIS FAITH IN ME, AND HELPED IN GUIDING ME TO A FULL HEALING. FINALLY, I WANT TO THANK MY FAMILY, FRIENDS AND ALL MY CHURCH FRIENDS FOR THEIR PRAYERS AND SUPPORT. EVEN THOUGH MANY OF THEM DIDN'T AGREE WITH MY DECISION, THEY NONETHELESS SUPPORTED ME WITHOUT EXCEPTION. SO A BIG THANKS TO ALL OF YOU!

ABOUT THE AUTHOR

John Marra has been a lifelong resident of Cleveland, Ohio. He's been married for 23 years and is a father of four and grandfather of twins.

Realizing after a second biopsy surgery that his cancer had returned with even more aggression, John decided to take matters into his own hands. He asked God for the Wisdom of Solomon to help him find a way to beat cancer. Turns out, God listened. John's story is about looking within oneself and realizing that the perfect running machine God gave us, our bodies, if given the chance, can heal itself.

Presently John runs a small business in Cleveland, Ohio called Marra's Market. He is willing to share with any customers who come to his store his journey that saved him succumbing to cancer.

YOU CAN READ MORE ABOUT JOHN MARRA
AND HIS JOURNEY AT:
HTTP://BEATBLADDERCANCER.BLOGSPOT.COM